INDEPENDENT STUDY GUIDE

HIMSS CAHIMS 2026

Study Guide 2026

✓ Aligned to official exam objectives
✓ Adversarially verified practice questions
✓ Complete preparation resource

Meridian Certification Press
An imprint of Big Five Killer

HIMSS CAHIMS 2026
Study Guide 2026

Published by Meridian Certification Press
An imprint of Big Five Killer

ISBN 9798259502444 (Paperback)
ISBN 9798259502468 (Hardcover)

AI Disclosure. Portions of this book were drafted with the assistance of large language models. All content was reviewed, edited, and verified by the editorial team at Meridian Certification Press. Practice questions and answer explanations underwent adversarial accuracy review.

Accuracy Commitment. If you believe you have found an error, please report it to `meridian@bigfivekiller.online`.

First edition, May 2026.

Contents

The complete revised study guide is written to `/tmp/cahims_2026_revised.md`. Here is the full revised document:

How to Use This Guide

This study guide is designed for candidates preparing for the HIMSS Certified Associate in Healthcare Information & Management Systems (CAHIMS) 2026 examination. CAHIMS is a foundational credential aimed at professionals new to the health informatics field — typically those with less than five years of full-time experience, recent graduates of health IT programs, or experienced clinicians and IT professionals transitioning into the healthcare informatics space.

0.1 Study Plan Recommendations

The CAHIMS exam tests breadth, not depth. Successful candidates report 60–120 hours of focused study over a 4- to 12-week window. Use the schedules in **Appendix C** to fit study time around work and family commitments. A typical week in the eight-week plan asks for 8–10 hours: roughly 3–4 hours of reading, 2–3 hours of practice questions, and 2–3 hours of review and weak-area drilling.

The exam blueprint (effective for 2026) covers six interrelated knowledge domains. Each chapter in this guide maps to one domain and includes:

- A statement of approximate exam weight so you can allocate study time proportionally.
- Three to five **learning objectives** stated as observable competencies, mirroring the way HIMSS frames blueprint tasks.
- Substantive content built around real workflows, standards (HL7, FHIR, IHE), and federal regulations (HIPAA, HITECH, 21st Century Cures, Information Blocking Rule).
- **Exam Tips** that highlight common test traps and high-yield facts.
- **Key Concepts** that summarize what HIMSS expects you to internalize.
- Five **Chapter Review Questions** modeled on the exam's multiple-choice, four-option format.

0.2 Practice Question Format

Every CAHIMS multiple-choice item presents a stem (a question or scenario) and exactly four answer options labeled A through D. Only one option is correct. Distractors are constructed to be plausible — they often state half-truths, swap roles (covered entity vs. business associate), or describe the right activity at the wrong stage of a systems lifecycle. Read the stem twice before reading any options, and treat "all of the above" or "none of the above" as red flags (HIMSS rarely uses them, but legacy banks may include them).

For each question in this guide, the answer is followed by a one- to two-sentence rationale that cites the relevant standard, regulation, or framework. Do not skip the rationales — they contain testable facts that may appear elsewhere in slightly different form.

0.3 Exam Day Tips

The exam is delivered through Pearson VUE at testing centers worldwide and via remote OnVUE proctoring. You will face 115 items (100 scored + 15 unscored pilot questions) and have two hours to complete them. That is roughly 62 seconds per question, so flag-and-return discipline matters.

- Bring two forms of government-issued ID. The name on each must match exactly the name on your registration.
- Arrive 30 minutes early. Late arrivals are usually rescheduled with a forfeit fee.
- Use the on-screen calculator only when arithmetic appears in a question; mental math is faster for the simple ratios CAHIMS uses.
- Use the **flag** feature for any item that requires more than 90 seconds. Finish the first pass, then return.
- Eliminate two wrong answers before guessing. The 25% baseline rises to 50% with two eliminations and ~67% with three.

Results — pass or fail — display on screen at the end of the session. A formal score report follows by email within five business days. The passing scaled score for CAHIMS is 70 on a 100-point scale. There is no penalty for incorrect answers; answer every question.

Healthcare Industry, Roles, and Stakeholders

Approximate Exam Weight: 15%

0.4 Learning Objectives

After completing this chapter, the candidate will be able to:

- Identify the major payer, provider, and regulatory stakeholders in the U.S. healthcare delivery system and describe their information-flow relationships.
- Explain the role of value-based purchasing programs (MIPS, ACO REACH, Hospital VBP) in driving health-IT investment.
- Distinguish among the principal accreditation, certification, and licensing bodies (CMS, ONC, The Joint Commission, NCQA, URAC) and the artifacts each produces.
- Map clinical workflows to the IT systems that support them across acute, ambulatory, post-acute, and home-care settings.

0.5 The U.S. Healthcare Delivery Landscape

The United States spent approximately $4.9 trillion on healthcare in 2023 (most recent finalized CMS National Health Expenditure data at the time of CAHIMS 2026 preparation; CMS published the 2023 NHE in December 2024, representing 17.6% of GDP). Preliminary CMS projections placed 2024 NHE at roughly $5.05 trillion. That spending flows through a four-sided system: **patients**, **providers**, **payers**, and **regulators**. Health IT sits at the intersection of all four. A CAHIMS candidate is expected to know who pays whom, who sets the rules, and which information system supports each transaction.

Patients consume care and increasingly act as data subjects with rights under HIPAA, the 21st Century Cures Act, and the Information Blocking Rule. Since the Cures Act final rule took full effect October 6, 2022, patients have a right to electronic access to all Electronic Health Information (EHI) in a designated record set without unreasonable delay and at no cost.

Providers include hospitals (about 6,100 in the U.S., per the American Hospital Association's 2024 fast facts), Critical Access Hospitals (CAHs, ≤25 beds, located in rural areas under the Medicare Rural Hospital Flexibility Program), Federally Qualified Health Centers (FQHCs) serving underserved populations, ambulatory practices, skilled nursing facilities (SNFs), home health agencies, hospices, and emerging telehealth-only organizations.

Payers finance care. The dominant federal payer is the Centers for Medicare & Medicaid Services (CMS), administering Medicare (Part A hospital, Part B physician, Part C Medicare Advantage, Part D prescription drug) and Medicaid (jointly administered with states). Commercial payers — UnitedHealthcare, Elevance Health (formerly Anthem), Aetna, Cigna, the Blue Cross Blue Shield Association plans, and Kaiser Permanente (integrated payer-provider) — cover most working-age Americans. The Veterans Health Administration, the Indian Health Service, and TRICARE round out the federal direct-care systems.

Regulators include CMS (Conditions of Participation), the Office of the National Coordinator for Health Information Technology (ONC, which certifies EHR technology), the Office for Civil Rights (OCR, which enforces HIPAA), the FDA (which regulates Software as a Medical Device, or SaMD, under the 21st Century Cures Act amendments to Section 520), and state Medicaid agencies and licensing boards. The Joint Commission, DNV Healthcare, and the Healthcare Facilities Accreditation Program (HFAP) are CMS-deemed accreditors for hospitals.

0.6 Value-Based Care and Health IT

For more than a decade, federal policy has shifted reimbursement from volume to value. CAHIMS candidates must understand the major programs because they drive system selection and configuration priorities.

The **Hospital Value-Based Purchasing (VBP) Program**, authorized by the Affordable Care Act § 3001, redistributes about 2% of inpatient prospective payment system (IPPS) Medicare payments based on quality and efficiency. Hospitals are measured on safety (CAUTI, CLABSI, CDI rates from NHSN reporting), clinical outcomes (30-day risk-standardized mortality for AMI, heart failure, pneumonia, COPD), person and community engagement (HCAHPS), and Medicare spending per beneficiary.

The **Merit-based Incentive Payment System (MIPS)**, the dominant Quality Payment Program track for eligible clinicians, scores participants across four categories: Quality (30%), Cost (30%), Improvement Activities (15%), and Promoting Interoperability (25%) for the 2026 performance period. The Promoting Interoperability category replaces the legacy Meaningful Use program and requires use of 2015 Edition Cures Update certified EHR technology.

The **ACO Realizing Equity, Access, and Community Health (REACH) Model**, which replaced the Direct Contracting Model in 2023, is one of several CMS Innovation Center accountable care arrangements. Both REACH and the Medicare Shared Savings Program (MSSP) require participants to manage attributed populations using risk-stratification, care-coordination workflows, and bidirectional data exchange with primary care, post-acute, and behavioral health partners.

0.7 Accreditation and Certification Bodies

Body	Scope	Key Artifact
The Joint Commission (TJC)	Hospitals, ambulatory, behavioral, home care	Comprehensive Accreditation Manual; National Patient Safety Goals
DNV Healthcare	Hospitals (deemed by CMS since 2008)	NIAHO standards
HFAP	Hospitals, ambulatory surgery	HFAP standards
NCQA	Health plans, PCMH, ACO, credentialing	HEDIS measures; PCMH recognition
URAC	Health plans, specialty pharmacy, telehealth	URAC accreditation modules
AAAHC	Ambulatory care	AAAHC handbook
HITRUST	Information security	HITRUST CSF
ONC	Health IT modules	ONC Health IT Certification Program, 2015 Edition Cures Update

For CAHIMS purposes, the most exam-relevant pairing is **ONC certifying technology** and **CMS attesting payment:** a clinician earns Promoting Interoperability credit only by using ONC-certified EHR technology that supports specific certification criteria (e.g., § 170.315(b)(1) Transitions of Care, § 170.315(g)(10) Standardized API for patient and population services).

0.8 Care Settings and the Systems That Support Them

A CAHIMS candidate should be able to map a care setting to the dominant clinical system and the data interfaces it requires.

- **Acute inpatient** — full Electronic Health Record (EHR), CPOE, eMAR, nursing flowsheets, ADT (Admission/Discharge/Transfer), interfaces to lab (LIS), radiology (RIS/PACS), and pharmacy.
- **Ambulatory** — EHR practice management bundle, patient portal, e-prescribing via Surescripts, and clinical quality measure (eCQM) reporting.
- **Emergency department** — ED information system (EDIS) integrated to the inpatient EHR; tracking board; disposition workflows.
- **Operating room** — Anesthesia Information Management System (AIMS), perioperative documentation, instrument and implant tracking.

- **Post-acute (SNF, IRF, LTCH)** — Minimum Data Set (MDS 3.0 for SNF) drives both clinical care plans and PDPM payment under Medicare; LTCH CARE Data Set drives PDPM-equivalent payment.
- **Home health and hospice** — OASIS-E1 (effective January 1, 2025) and HIS data submission to CMS; point-of-care mobile documentation.
- **Behavioral health** — separate EHR or behavioral module with stricter consent (42 CFR Part 2 governs substance use disorder records).

> **Exam Tip**
>
> When a question mentions 42 CFR Part 2, think substance use disorder records and a higher consent bar than HIPAA — patients must affirmatively authorize most disclosures of Part 2 records, even for treatment.

> **Exam Tip**
>
> Distinguish *certified* (ONC) from *accredited* (TJC, DNV, NCQA). EHRs are certified; organizations are accredited; individuals are credentialed.

> **Exam Tip**
>
> The 21st Century Cures Act prohibits **information blocking** by actors (providers, HIEs/HINs, and developers of certified health IT). Civil monetary penalties for developers can reach $1 million per violation under OIG regulations finalized in 2023.

> **Key Concept**
>
> Value-based care reimbursement rewards outcomes and total cost of care; it is the principal financial driver for interoperability, quality reporting, and population health IT investments.

> **Key Concept**
>
> Health IT lives between the four corners of the system — patients, providers, payers, regulators — and every system selection should be justified by which of those relationships it enables.

> **Key Concept**
>
> Certification and accreditation are distinct: ONC certifies *technology*, CMS-deemed bodies accredit *organizations*, and state boards license *individuals*.

0.9 Chapter 1 Review Questions

Q1. A community hospital wants its physicians to earn full credit in the MIPS Promoting Interoperability category for the 2026 performance period. Which technology requirement must it meet?

A) Use of any EHR system currently in production.
B) Use of EHR technology certified to the 2015 Edition Cures Update.
C) Use of an EHR vendor on the CMS preferred-vendor list.
D) Use of a HITRUST CSF–certified EHR vendor.

Answer: B — MIPS Promoting Interoperability requires the use of 2015 Edition Cures Update certified EHR technology meeting specific § 170.315 criteria; there is no CMS preferred-vendor list, and HITRUST is a separate security framework.

Q2. Which federal law established the patient's right to receive Electronic Health Information without unreasonable delay and prohibited information blocking by providers and developers?

A) HIPAA Privacy Rule (1996)
B) HITECH Act (2009)
C) 21st Century Cures Act (2016)
D) Affordable Care Act (2010)

Answer: C — The 21st Century Cures Act, signed in December 2016, established the information blocking provisions and the right to EHI access. The ONC and OIG final rules implementing it took effect in 2020–2023.

Q3. A Skilled Nursing Facility's clinical documentation system must support which CMS-required data set to drive both care planning and PDPM payment?

A) OASIS-E1
B) MDS 3.0
C) IRF-PAI
D) UB-04

Answer: B — The Minimum Data Set (MDS) 3.0 is the resident assessment instrument SNFs use; OASIS-E1 is home health, IRF-PAI is inpatient rehab, and UB-04 is an institutional billing form.

Q4. Records covered under 42 CFR Part 2 are subject to a stricter consent standard than HIPAA. These records pertain to:

A) Behavioral health services in any setting
B) Substance use disorder treatment provided by federally assisted programs
C) HIV/AIDS testing and treatment
D) Genetic testing results

Answer: B — 42 CFR Part 2 governs substance use disorder records held by federally assisted programs. The 2024 final rule aligned Part 2 more closely with HIPAA but retained heightened patient-consent requirements.

Q5. A hospital seeking CMS-deemed status may choose among several accrediting bodies. Which of the following is a CMS-deemed hospital accreditor?

A) NCQA
B) URAC
C) DNV Healthcare
D) AAAHC

Answer: C — DNV Healthcare (NIAHO standards) has held CMS deeming authority for hospitals since 2008. NCQA accredits health plans, URAC accredits health plans and specialty pharmacy, and AAAHC accredits ambulatory care.

Technology Environment

Approximate Exam Weight: 20%

0.10 Learning Objectives

After completing this chapter, the candidate will be able to:

- Describe the hardware, networking, virtualization, and cloud-deployment models used in modern healthcare IT environments.
- Identify the principal interoperability standards (HL7 v2, HL7 CDA, HL7 FHIR R4, DICOM, NCPDP SCRIPT, X12 270/271/278/835/837) and the use cases each supports.
- Explain core terminologies and code sets (ICD-10-CM/PCS, CPT, HCPCS, SNOMED CT, LOINC, RxNorm) and where each appears in clinical workflow.
- Apply common networking and integration patterns — integration engines, APIs, HIE/HIN, and TEFCA QHIN exchange.
- Recognize the key 2023–2026 federal interoperability rulemakings (ONC HTI-1, CMS Interoperability and Prior Authorization, ASTP/ONC HTI-2) and their implications for health-IT compliance dates.

0.11 Hardware, Virtualization, and Cloud

Hospital data centers historically ran on x86 servers in rack-mounted form, with redundant power, cooling, and dual storage area networks (SAN) for the EHR. The dominant pattern in 2026 is hybrid: production workloads remain in vendor-hosted data centers (Epic Hosted, Oracle Health Hosted, MEDITECH Cloud), with analytics, AI, and disaster recovery in the public cloud (AWS, Microsoft Azure, Google Cloud Platform). Smaller ambulatory practices have largely moved to fully cloud-hosted EHRs (athenaOne, eClinicalWorks Cloud).

A CAHIMS candidate should understand the three cloud service models:

- **Infrastructure as a Service (IaaS)** — raw compute, storage, and networking (AWS EC2, Azure Virtual Machines). The customer manages OS, middleware, and applications.
- **Platform as a Service (PaaS)** — managed runtime, databases, and developer tools (Azure App Service, Google App Engine). The customer manages applications and data.
- **Software as a Service (SaaS)** — fully managed applications delivered over the web (athenaOne, Microsoft 365). The customer manages only configuration and data.

And the four deployment models — public, private, community, and hybrid — defined in NIST SP 800-145.

Under HIPAA, any cloud service provider that creates, receives, maintains, or transmits Protected Health Information (PHI) on behalf of a covered entity is a **business associate** and must execute a Business Associate Agreement (BAA). This applies even when the data is encrypted and the provider has no theoretical access to it (OCR's October 2016 cloud computing guidance).

0.12 Networking Fundamentals for Health IT

Healthcare networks blend wired clinical workstations, Wi-Fi mobile carts (WoWs), barcode scanners, telemetry, biomedical devices, and increasingly Internet-of-Medical-Things (IoMT) infusion pumps and patient monitors. The CAHIMS exam tests fundamentals — the OSI model, TCP/IP, DNS, DHCP, and VPN basics — rather than deep network engineering.

Key concepts:

- **VLAN segmentation** — biomedical devices on separate VLANs from clinical workstations limit lateral movement during a ransomware incident.
- **Wi-Fi 6 / Wi-Fi 6E (802.11ax)** — standard in new hospital builds; supports the density required by mobile carts and patient-owned devices on guest SSIDs.

- **VPN and Zero Trust** — clinicians working remotely connect through SSL/IPsec VPN or, increasingly, through Zero Trust Network Access (ZTNA) brokers that authenticate every session and device.
- **Bandwidth and latency** — DICOM imaging and high-acuity telehealth drive bandwidth; tele-ICU and remote robotic surgery drive latency requirements (often <100 ms round trip).

0.13 Interoperability Standards

CAHIMS candidates must know what each standard does, not how to implement it.

HL7 Version 2.x (v2.5.1 is the most widely deployed) — pipe-and-hat delimited messages for ADT, ORM (orders), ORU (results), MDM (documents), and SIU (scheduling). v2 messages flow over Minimum Lower Layer Protocol (MLLP) through integration engines (Rhapsody, Mirth/NextGen Connect, Cloverleaf, Iguana, Corepoint).

HL7 CDA (Clinical Document Architecture) Release 2 — XML-based clinical documents. The **Consolidated CDA (C-CDA) Release 2.1** templates implement Continuity of Care Document (CCD), Discharge Summary, and the **U.S. Core Data for Interoperability (USCDI)** v4 (the version current for ONC 2026 certification).

HL7 FHIR Release 4 (R4) — RESTful API standard using JSON or XML. The ONC 2015 Cures Update certification criterion § 170.315(g)(10) historically required Standardized API access using FHIR R4, the SMART App Launch 1.0 framework with the v1.0 OAuth 2.0 scopes, and the US Core 3.1.1 Implementation Guide. Per the ONC HTI-1 Final Rule (December 2023), the (g)(10) baseline is being updated through phased compliance dates referencing USCDI v3 with newer US Core versions. Candidates should know US Core 3.1.1 as the historical minimum and US Core 6.1.0 (or later) as the current direction under HTI-1's phased schedule. FHIR R5 was published in 2023 but is not yet the regulated version for (g)(10).

DICOM (Digital Imaging and Communications in Medicine) — the standard for medical imaging, governing both wire format and the Service-Object Pair (SOP) classes that define operations (C-STORE, C-FIND, C-MOVE). All PACS systems speak DICOM.

NCPDP SCRIPT — the e-prescribing standard, used over the Surescripts network for new prescriptions, refills, change requests, cancellation, and (since 2018) electronic prior authorization.

X12 transactions, mandated by HIPAA, support administrative workflows: - 270/271 eligibility inquiry and response - 276/277 claim status inquiry and response - 278 services review (prior authorization) - 834 enrollment - 835 electronic remittance advice - 837 healthcare claim (P professional, I institutional, D dental)

IHE (Integrating the Healthcare Enterprise) profiles package these standards into reusable workflows — for example, IHE XDS.b (Cross-Enterprise Document Sharing) and IHE PIX/PDQ (patient identification).

0.14 Terminologies and Code Sets

Standard	Domain	Maintained By
ICD-10-CM	Diagnoses (U.S.)	NCHS
ICD-10-PCS	Inpatient procedures	CMS
CPT	Outpatient procedures, E&M	AMA
HCPCS Level II	Supplies, DME, drugs	CMS
SNOMED CT	Clinical concepts	SNOMED International (NLM is U.S. release center)
LOINC	Lab and clinical observations	Regenstrief Institute
RxNorm	Clinical drugs	NLM
UCUM	Units of measure	Regenstrief Institute
CVX/MVX	Vaccines / manufacturers	CDC

USCDI v4 (published July 2023, mandatory for ONC certification in 2026) explicitly requires SNOMED CT for problems, LOINC for laboratory observations, and RxNorm for medications. CPT and ICD-10-CM remain the financial code sets but are not part of USCDI.

0.15 ONC HTI-1 Final Rule and Decision Support Interventions

The **ONC HTI-1 Final Rule** (published December 13, 2023, effective in stages through 2025–2026) introduces the **Decision Support Interventions (DSI) certification criterion at § 170.315(b)(11)**, which replaces the prior Clinical Decision Support (CDS) criterion. The DSI criterion is highly relevant to 2026 exam currency on AI/CDS transparency.

Under § 170.315(b)(11), certified health IT must support two types of decision support:

- **Evidence-based DSIs** — interventions based on clinical knowledge (guidelines, literature) that act on patient data.
- **Predictive DSIs** — models that produce outputs derived from algorithms or statistical methods (including AI/ML).

For **predictive DSIs**, certified health IT must make accessible to users a set of **source attributes**, including:

1. Description and intended use of the intervention.
2. Intended user(s).
3. Cautioned, out-of-scope, or otherwise inappropriate uses.
4. Training data description.
5. Performance metrics (validation, fairness/bias evaluation).
6. Identification of inputs (variables, features).
7. Output description.
8. Quantitative measures of performance.
9. External validation processes.
10. Approach to ongoing monitoring and update management.

HTI-1 also imposes an **insights condition for certification**, requiring developers to publish information on real-world use and performance of certified DSIs. Together with the **USCDI v3 transition timeline**, HTI-1 reshapes the (g)(10) baseline and the transparency expectations for clinical AI.

0.16 CMS Interoperability and Prior Authorization Final Rule (January 2024)

The **CMS Interoperability and Prior Authorization Final Rule** (CMS-0057-F), published January 17, 2024, applies to Medicare Advantage organizations, Medicaid and CHIP fee-for-service programs and managed care plans, and qualified health plan issuers on the Federally-facilitated Exchanges. It requires impacted payers to:

- **Patient Access API** — expand the existing FHIR-based Patient Access API to include information about prior authorization decisions.
- **Provider Access API** — implement a FHIR-based API enabling providers to retrieve patient data for treatment purposes (effective January 1, 2027).
- **Payer-to-Payer API** — implement a FHIR-based API enabling exchange of patient data between payers when a member changes plans (effective January 1, 2027).
- **Prior Authorization API** — implement a FHIR-based API supporting CRD (Coverage Requirements Discovery), DTR (Documentation Templates and Rules), and PAS (Prior Authorization Support) for electronic prior authorization (effective January 1, 2027).

Compliance with prior authorization decision timeframes (72 hours for expedited, 7 calendar days for standard) begins January 1, 2026, with API requirements effective January 1, 2027.

0.17 ASTP/ONC HTI-2 Proposed Rule (2024)

ONC was rebranded the **Assistant Secretary for Technology Policy (ASTP)** in 2024 while continuing to administer ONC certification programs. ASTP/ONC published the **HTI-2 Proposed Rule** in 2024, extending interoperability requirements to public health reporting workflows and adding new certification criteria for payer-provider FHIR exchange (case reporting, electronic laboratory reporting, immunization administration, syndromic surveillance, and other public health use cases). Candidates should recognize HTI-2 by name and broad scope; specific compliance dates were not yet finalized as of early 2026.

0.18 Integration Engines, APIs, and HIE/HIN/TEFCA

Most hospitals route HL7 v2 traffic through a centralized **integration engine** that performs message transformation, routing, persistence for replay, and acknowledgement handling. The engine isolates source systems from changes downstream.

For external exchange, three patterns dominate in 2026:

1. **Direct Secure Messaging** — SMTP-based secure email with S/MIME encryption, between Direct Trust–accredited HISPs. Still used for transitions of care and provider-to-provider messaging.
2. **Health Information Exchanges (HIEs) and Health Information Networks (HINs)** — regional (e.g., CRISP in Maryland) or national networks (CommonWell, Carequality) that broker query-based document exchange using IHE XDS.b/XCA.
3. **TEFCA Qualified Health Information Networks (QHINs)** — under the **Trusted Exchange Framework and Common Agreement** finalized by ONC in January 2022 and operational since 2023, designated QHINs provide a single on-ramp for cross-network exchange. The first five QHINs were designated in December 2023 (eHealth Exchange, Epic Nexus, Health Gorilla, KONZA, and MedAllies), with additional QHINs (including CommonWell in February 2024) added through 2024 and 2025. Participants connect to a QHIN once and reach every other QHIN's network.

> **Exam Tip**
>
> When a question contrasts HL7 v2 and FHIR, remember: v2 is messaging (push, MLLP), FHIR is API (pull or push, REST/JSON). They are complementary, not competing — a modern hospital runs both.

> **Exam Tip**
>
> Cloud providers that touch PHI are business associates **even when the data is encrypted end-to-end**; OCR's 2016 guidance is explicit on this. Always require a BAA.

> **Exam Tip**
>
> When you see "USCDI" in a stem, think of it as the *content* standard (what data must be exchanged), and FHIR R4 / C-CDA as the *transport and structure* standards (how it is exchanged).

> **Exam Tip**
>
> The HTI-1 Final Rule (December 2023) introduced the DSI criterion at § 170.315(b)(11). When a question references "Decision Support Interventions" or "predictive DSI source attributes," HTI-1 is the answer.

> **Key Concept**
>
> Standards classify by purpose: messaging (HL7 v2, NCPDP SCRIPT), documents (CDA, C-CDA), APIs (FHIR), imaging (DICOM), administrative (X12), and terminology (SNOMED, LOINC, RxNorm, ICD-10, CPT).

> **Key Concept**
>
> TEFCA is not a network — it is an agreement framework that makes participating networks interoperable through designated QHINs.

> **Key Concept**
>
> Hybrid cloud is the dominant deployment model for U.S. hospitals in 2026; the BAA, not the deployment model, is what determines HIPAA compliance posture.

> **Key Concept**
>
> The 2023–2024 federal interoperability rulemakings — ONC HTI-1 (DSI criterion, USCDI v3 transition) and CMS Interoperability and Prior Authorization (Patient/Provider/Payer-to-Payer/Prior Authorization APIs) — set the 2026–2027 compliance horizon.

0.19 Chapter 2 Review Questions

Q1. Which interoperability standard is required by the ONC 2015 Edition Cures Update § 170.315(g)(10) Standardized API certification criterion?

A) HL7 v2.5.1 over MLLP
B) HL7 CDA Release 2
C) HL7 FHIR Release 4 with US Core Implementation Guide and SMART App Launch
D) DICOM SOP Class C-STORE

Answer: C — The (g)(10) criterion requires FHIR R4, US Core (3.1.1 historically; 6.1.0+ under HTI-1's phased schedule), and SMART App Launch 1.0 with the v1 OAuth 2.0 scopes for patient and population services.

Q2. A health system contracts with a cloud vendor to host its data warehouse. The data warehouse contains de-identified analytics extracts and re-identification keys held by a separate covered-entity custodian. Under HIPAA, what agreement does the vendor require?

A) None, because the data is de-identified.
B) A Business Associate Agreement, because it creates, receives, maintains, or transmits PHI on behalf of a covered entity.
C) A Data Use Agreement only.
D) A standard cloud service contract.

Answer: B — Because the dataset can be re-identified using a key held by a covered entity, the cloud vendor is handling PHI on behalf of the covered entity and is a business associate. OCR's 2016 cloud guidance also clarifies that even ciphertext-only providers must execute BAAs.

Q3. Which terminology is the USCDI-required standard for laboratory observation identifiers?

A) SNOMED CT
B) LOINC
C) RxNorm
D) ICD-10-CM

Answer: B — LOINC (Logical Observation Identifiers Names and Codes), maintained by the Regenstrief Institute, is the USCDI-mandated terminology for laboratory and other observations.

Q4. A radiology PACS sends a study to an outside reading service using DICOM. Which DICOM service class describes the transfer of a complete imaging study to a remote node?

A) C-FIND
B) C-MOVE
C) C-STORE
D) C-ECHO

Answer: C — C-STORE transmits a Composite SOP Instance (image) to a remote application entity. C-FIND queries, C-MOVE coordinates a transfer, and C-ECHO is a verification ping.

Q5. Under TEFCA, a hospital that wants to query patient records across the country must:

A) Connect directly to every other hospital's API individually.
B) Connect to a designated Qualified Health Information Network (QHIN).
C) Use only Direct Secure Messaging.
D) Submit a request to the Office of the National Coordinator.

Answer: B — TEFCA designates QHINs as the on-ramp; a participant connects to one QHIN and exchanges with all other QHINs and their participants through the Common Agreement.

Systems Analysis, Design, and Selection

Approximate Exam Weight: 20%

0.20 Learning Objectives

After completing this chapter, the candidate will be able to:

- Describe the phases of the Systems Development Life Cycle (SDLC) and identify deliverables at each phase.
- Conduct or contribute to clinical and operational workflow analysis using accepted modeling tools.
- Develop functional and non-functional requirements that support an objective system selection.
- Apply structured vendor evaluation methods (RFI, RFP, demos, reference checks, total cost of ownership).

0.21 The Systems Development Life Cycle

The SDLC is the umbrella framework HIMSS uses to organize the analysis, design, build, test, deploy, and maintain activities. Two variants matter for CAHIMS:

Waterfall — sequential phases with formal gates: Planning □ Analysis □ Design □ Build □ Test □ Implement □ Operate & Maintain. Waterfall predominates in EHR core builds because regulatory and clinical safety needs argue for documented, gated decisions.

Agile / iterative — short sprints (typically two to four weeks) producing working increments of functionality. Agile predominates in custom application development, integration work, and population health analytics builds. Hybrid (Agile build inside a Waterfall implementation contract) is the practical norm for EHR optimization.

A CAHIMS candidate should know typical deliverables at each phase:

Phase	Typical Deliverables
Planning	Project charter, scope statement, high-level budget and timeline
Analysis	Workflow diagrams, requirements document, gap analysis
Design	Functional design specs, technical design specs, data model
Build	Configured system, custom code, integrations
Test	Test plans, unit/integration/UAT scripts, defect log
Implement	Cutover plan, training materials, go-live support model
Operate	Runbooks, optimization backlog, SLA reporting

0.22 Workflow Analysis

Workflow analysis precedes both selection and configuration. Good analysis prevents the most common implementation failure: paving an inefficient paper workflow into the EHR. Standard modeling tools include:

- **Swimlane / cross-functional flowchart** — roles on the Y-axis, time on the X-axis, decision diamonds for branching. This is the most testable workflow notation on CAHIMS.
- **BPMN (Business Process Model and Notation) 2.0** — formal modeling for IT-led process redesign.
- **Value Stream Map (VSM)** — Lean technique that distinguishes value-added from non-value-added time; useful for ED throughput, OR turnover, and revenue cycle analysis.
- **Use case / user story** — Agile-style "As a [role], I want [feature] so that [benefit]" format.

When performing analysis, the analyst observes the **current state** (As-Is), then designs the **future state** (To-Be). The gap between the two is the requirements set.

0.23 Requirements: Functional vs. Non-Functional

Functional requirements describe what the system must *do*. Examples: "The CPOE module shall display drug-drug interactions of severity level 2 or higher at order entry." Functional requirements drive vendor scoring on RFP responses.

Non-functional requirements (NFRs) describe how the system must perform. Common NFR categories:

- **Performance** — page load <2 seconds, batch job runtime <4 hours.
- **Availability** — 99.95% uptime (≈4.4 hours of downtime per year).
- **Scalability** — supports 5,000 concurrent users.
- **Security** — supports SAML 2.0 SSO, AES-256 encryption at rest, TLS 1.3 in transit.
- **Usability** — task completion within X clicks; SUS score ≥75.
- **Maintainability** — vendor-supported configuration, no custom code lock-in.
- **Compliance** — ONC 2015 Edition Cures Update certified.

NFRs are frequently overlooked in selection but cause most post–go-live regret.

0.24 Vendor Selection: RFI, RFP, Demo, Reference

A typical large EHR or revenue cycle selection follows a multi-stage funnel:

1. **Request for Information (RFI)** — broad, qualitative; identifies a short list of viable vendors. Open-ended questions about capabilities and roadmap.
2. **Request for Proposal (RFP)** — detailed, often hundreds of requirements scored by the buyer. Vendors commit pricing and contractual terms. CAHIMS candidates should expect questions distinguishing RFI (information gathering) from RFP (binding proposal).
3. **Scripted demonstration** — vendors demonstrate the same clinical scenarios on the buyer's behalf. The script is written by the buyer to ensure apples-to-apples comparison.
4. **Reference checks and site visits** — buyer speaks to peer customers of similar size, complexity, and integration profile. Visit a live customer site to observe actual clinical use, not the showroom.
5. **Total Cost of Ownership (TCO) analysis** — five- to seven-year window covering software license, implementation services, infrastructure, internal labor, training, integration, ongoing maintenance and support, and end-of-life or replacement.

A vendor scoring matrix typically weights requirements by criticality: must-have (1.0), should-have (0.7), nice-to-have (0.3). The lowest-cost vendor rarely wins; the best total value typically does.

0.25 Contracts and Risk Management

A CAHIMS candidate should recognize, but not draft, the following contract artifacts:

- **Master Services Agreement (MSA)** with **Statements of Work (SOWs)** for implementation services.
- **Software License Agreement** with named-user, concurrent-user, or enterprise license terms.
- **Service Level Agreement (SLA)** specifying uptime, response, and resolution targets with financial credits for missed levels.
- **Business Associate Agreement (BAA)** — mandatory whenever the vendor will touch PHI.
- **Source code escrow** — protects the customer if the vendor goes bankrupt; less common with major EHRs.
- **Indemnification and limitation of liability** — limits one party's exposure for the other's wrongdoing; HIPAA-related claims are typically carved out.

> **Exam Tip**
>
> "Total Cost of Ownership" is the right answer when a question asks how to compare two systems that have very different up-front prices and ongoing fees.

> **Exam Tip**
>
> If a question contrasts RFI and RFP, RFI is exploratory (no binding pricing), RFP is procurement (binding pricing and terms).

> **Exam Tip**
>
> The phrase "non-functional requirement" appears in CAHIMS exam stems; remember that performance, availability, scalability, security, and usability are all non-functional, even though they are essential.

> **Key Concept**
>
> Workflow analysis is the prerequisite to configuration. Paving paper inefficiency into the EHR is the canonical implementation failure mode.

> **Key Concept**
>
> SDLC phases — Plan, Analyze, Design, Build, Test, Implement, Operate — each have specific deliverables that gate the next phase.

> **Key Concept**
>
> A vendor scoring matrix should weight requirements (must/should/nice) and combine functional capability with TCO and risk to produce a defensible decision.

0.26 Chapter 3 Review Questions

Q1. A health system is comparing three EHR vendors. Two have low initial license fees but high annual maintenance and integration costs; the third has high initial fees but bundled support. Which analytical tool best supports an apples-to-apples comparison?

A) Net Present Value of license fees alone
B) Total Cost of Ownership over a seven-year horizon
C) Vendor reference scores
D) Scripted demonstration outcomes

Answer: B — TCO across a multi-year horizon (typically five to seven years) is the correct framework, because it captures license, maintenance, integration, infrastructure, internal labor, and replacement costs.

Q2. Which of the following is a non-functional requirement?

A) The CPOE shall present drug-drug interactions at order entry.
B) The patient portal shall allow patients to schedule appointments.
C) The EHR shall achieve 99.95% availability measured monthly.
D) The lab module shall accept HL7 ORU R01 result messages.

Answer: C — Availability targets are classic non-functional requirements. The other three describe what the system does (functional).

Q3. During system selection, a hospital sends out a 400-question document with binding pricing requested and a deadline for response. This document is a:

A) Request for Information
B) Request for Proposal
C) Statement of Work
D) Master Services Agreement

Answer: B — A binding RFP with detailed requirements and pricing is the procurement document. An RFI is exploratory and non-binding.

Q4. A clinical informaticist diagrams the current ED triage process showing nurse, registrar, and physician activities along a timeline with handoffs and decision points. Which workflow modeling technique is being used?

A) Value Stream Map
B) Swimlane diagram
C) Use case diagram
D) Entity-Relationship diagram

Answer: B — A swimlane diagram shows roles as lanes and the process flow across them; it is the most common workflow modeling tool in healthcare SDLC analysis.

Q5. Which contract artifact is *mandatory* between a covered entity and any vendor that creates, receives, maintains, or transmits PHI?

A) Master Services Agreement
B) Service Level Agreement
C) Business Associate Agreement
D) Source Code Escrow

Answer: C — The HIPAA Privacy and Security Rules require a written Business Associate Agreement before PHI can be disclosed to a business associate.

System Implementation, Support, and Maintenance

Approximate Exam Weight: 15%

0.27 Learning Objectives

After completing this chapter, the candidate will be able to:

- Plan and execute the principal activities of an EHR or ancillary system implementation: build, test, train, convert data, and cut over.
- Distinguish among cutover strategies (big bang, phased rollout, parallel, pilot) and select an appropriate strategy for a given context.
- Identify the IT service management processes — incident, problem, change, release, and configuration management — that govern post–go-live operations.
- Plan and execute system upgrades, optimization initiatives, and decommissioning.
- Recognize the relationship between health-IT–related sentinel events and The Joint Commission's Sentinel Event Policy.

0.28 Implementation Phases

After a contract is signed, the implementation phase begins. Major activities run in parallel:

Build — configuring the system to the organization's workflows. For an EHR, this includes order set development, smart text and notes templates, security roles, document routing, and clinical decision support rule activation. Build is typically organized by analyst team aligned to clinical domain (ED, inpatient, ambulatory, ancillary).

Integration build — interface engineers configure HL7 v2 routes, FHIR endpoints, and (where the vendor supports them) IHE profiles to and from ancillary systems. Each interface is documented in an interface specification.

Data conversion — historical data is migrated from legacy systems. A reasonable approach is to convert structured data critical to current care (allergies, medications, problems, immunizations) and reference legacy charts for everything else. Full conversion of years of free-text notes is rarely worth the cost.

Training — typically structured as role-based curricula. Most large EHR vendors require credentialed trainers and provide a "train the trainer" model. Training intensity ranges from four to twenty-four hours depending on role and system complexity.

Testing — at minimum: unit testing (single function), integration testing (interfaces and dependent systems), system testing (end-to-end clinical scenarios), user acceptance testing (UAT, with clinical end users), and parallel testing where dual-system operation is feasible. A common test management tool maps each requirement to one or more test scripts.

Cutover planning — defines the freeze date for legacy system changes, the data-extraction sequence, the activation steps, the rollback criteria, and the at-the-elbow support model for the first 24–72 hours.

0.29 Cutover Strategies

Strategy	Description	When to Use	Risks
Big bang	All locations, all modules cut over on a single date	Single hospital, integrated EHR	High risk, requires intensive command center

Strategy	Description	When to Use	Risks
Phased rollout	Modules or locations cut over sequentially	Multi-hospital system	Long dual-state period, integration complexity
Parallel	Old and new systems run side by side	Critical financial systems	Doubles work for staff
Pilot	One unit or clinic adopts first	Ambulatory rollouts	Pilot site may not represent the system

The dominant pattern for large hospital EHR go-lives is a **wave-based phased rollout** — typically 3 to 7 hospitals per wave, 6 to 12 weeks apart, with a command center, "at-the-elbow" superusers per unit, and a clinical optimization backlog scrubbed weekly.

0.30 ITIL and IT Service Management

After go-live, the work shifts from project to operations. CAHIMS draws heavily from the **ITIL 4** service management framework. Candidates should know the principal practices by what each does:

- **Incident management** — restore service after an unplanned interruption. A printer not working is an incident; the SLA defines target time to restore.
- **Problem management** — identify and remove the root cause of one or more incidents. Problem management is investigative; incident management is reactive.
- **Change management** — control changes to production. The Change Advisory Board (CAB) reviews change requests for risk, scheduling conflicts, and approvals. Categories typically include standard (pre-approved), normal (CAB-reviewed), and emergency (post-implementation review).
- **Release management** — package multiple changes into coordinated releases. EHR vendors typically deliver quarterly upgrades that customers schedule into their release calendar.
- **Configuration management** — maintain accurate inventory of components (CIs) in a Configuration Management Database (CMDB) so that change impact can be assessed.
- **Service request management** — handle user requests (access provisioning, password resets, report requests) distinct from incidents.

A **Service Level Agreement (SLA)** sets targets for incident response and resolution. Common severity tiers:

- Severity 1 — system down, patient safety risk; response within 15 minutes, restore within 4 hours.
- Severity 2 — major function impaired; response within 1 hour, restore within 8 hours.
- Severity 3 — minor function impaired; response within 4 hours, restore within 2 business days.
- Severity 4 — cosmetic or enhancement; scheduled.

0.31 Health-IT–Related Sentinel Events

The Joint Commission's **Sentinel Event Policy** defines a **sentinel event** as a patient safety event (not primarily related to the natural course of the patient's illness or underlying condition) that reaches a patient and results in death, permanent harm, or severe temporary harm. Reviewable sentinel events include, among others, suicide of a patient receiving care in a staffed-around-the-clock setting, surgery on the wrong patient or wrong site, retention of a foreign object, and severe medication errors.

Health-IT–related sentinel events are a recognized subset. Examples include:

- **Wrong-patient EHR errors** — clinician documents or orders on the wrong patient due to chart-selection ambiguity, simultaneous chart open in another tab, or barcode/printout mismatch.
- **CPOE misorders** — drug-drug interaction or allergy alerts overridden inappropriately, leading to harm.
- **Decision support failure** — CDS rule incorrectly suppressed by a build error or override-by-default behavior.
- **Interface failure with clinical consequence** — lab result not routed to the ordering provider; a critical value not flagged.

Joint Commission–accredited organizations are expected (but not required) to self-report sentinel events; when an event is reported, the organization must complete a **comprehensive systematic analysis** (root cause analysis) and submit a corrective action plan within 55 business days. Health IT teams are increasingly central participants in these analyses, and HIT-specific safety frameworks (ONC's SAFER Guides) are widely used for prospective risk assessment.

0.32 Upgrades, Optimization, and Decommissioning

EHR and ancillary system **upgrades** typically arrive on a quarterly or semi-annual cycle. Each upgrade goes through:

1. Vendor release-notes review
2. Build in a non-production environment (TEST or POC)
3. Regression test of in-scope workflows
4. Communication and training on new features
5. Production deployment in a scheduled change window
6. Post-deployment monitoring

Optimization is the steady stream of enhancement requests that follows any major go-live. A governance committee — often called a Clinical Informatics Council or Optimization Steering Committee — prioritizes the backlog using a scoring framework (impact, effort, regulatory required).

Decommissioning of legacy systems requires:

- Data retention plan aligned with HIPAA, state record retention statutes (commonly 7–10 years from last encounter, but varies), and Conditions of Participation.
- Migration of needed historical data to the new system or a long-term archive.
- Read-only access for clinicians for a defined period (often 12–24 months) before final shutoff.
- Secure destruction of media per NIST SP 800-88 Rev. 1 (Clear, Purge, Destroy).

> **Exam Tip**
>
> Incident management restores service. Problem management investigates root cause. CAHIMS frequently tests this distinction.

> **Exam Tip**
>
> A "big bang" cutover is not the same as "all at once." Big bang means all modules at one location on one date. Multi-hospital systems can still do a big bang per hospital while phasing across the system.

> **Exam Tip**
>
> When a stem mentions a Change Advisory Board, the topic is **change management**.

> **Exam Tip**
>
> When a stem describes a wrong-patient documentation error or a CDS-override harm event, think Joint Commission Sentinel Event Policy and ONC SAFER Guides.

> **Key Concept**
>
> Implementation success depends on disciplined build, testing, training, conversion, and cutover; each can sink the project if neglected.

> **Key Concept**
>
> ITIL 4 practices (incident, problem, change, release, configuration) structure post–go-live operations and are the most common source of CAHIMS questions about IT service management.

> **Key Concept**
> Legacy system decommissioning is governed by federal and state retention statutes plus organizational policy; secure media disposal follows NIST SP 800-88 Rev. 1.

0.33 Chapter 4 Review Questions

Q1. A nurse calls the IT service desk to report that the medication administration system stopped scanning barcodes house-wide. The service desk creates a ticket and immediately escalates. Which ITIL practice describes the activity of restoring barcode scanning service as quickly as possible?
A) Problem management
B) Change management
C) Incident management
D) Configuration management

Answer: C — Incident management focuses on restoring normal service operation as quickly as possible after an unplanned interruption. Problem management would investigate the root cause after service is restored.

Q2. A health system plans to migrate from a legacy lab system to a new vendor's LIS. Which decommissioning activity is governed by NIST SP 800-88 Revision 1?
A) Negotiating the vendor contract
B) Sanitizing storage media after data migration
C) Performing the cutover
D) Training the staff on the new system

Answer: B — NIST SP 800-88 Rev. 1 provides guidance on media sanitization, defining Clear, Purge, and Destroy categories for end-of-life storage media.

Q3. A six-hospital system is implementing a new EHR. Each hospital cuts over individually, six weeks apart, with all modules going live together at each site. This is best described as:
A) Big bang across the system
B) Phased rollout with per-site big bang activations
C) Parallel implementation
D) Pilot implementation

Answer: B — Sequential per-site activations constitute a phased rollout, even though each site experiences a big-bang go-live for its modules.

Q4. During UAT, end users discover that the medication reconciliation workflow does not match a state Board of Pharmacy requirement that becomes effective the day after go-live. What is the appropriate response?
A) Delay go-live indefinitely.
B) Document the gap, score its severity, and decide whether to remediate before go-live or as a post–go-live optimization.
C) Ignore the gap because UAT is for usability only.
D) Cancel UAT and restart system selection.

Answer: B — UAT exists to surface gaps. The appropriate response is structured defect triage that weighs regulatory risk against schedule and cost.

Q5. Which ITIL artifact maintains an accurate inventory of components and their relationships so that the impact of a proposed change can be assessed?
A) Change schedule
B) Service catalog
C) Configuration Management Database (CMDB)
D) Known error database

Answer: C — The CMDB inventories configuration items (CIs) and their relationships, enabling change impact assessment.

Information Privacy and Security

Approximate Exam Weight: 15%

0.34 Learning Objectives

After completing this chapter, the candidate will be able to:

- Apply the HIPAA Privacy, Security, and Breach Notification Rules to common health-IT scenarios.
- Identify administrative, physical, and technical safeguards from 45 CFR Part 164 Subpart C and map them to organizational controls.
- Recognize the principal cybersecurity threats to healthcare (ransomware, phishing, BEC, supply-chain compromise, medical-device exploitation) and the controls that mitigate them.
- Conduct or contribute to security risk analysis and risk management activities consistent with NIST SP 800-30 / SP 800-66 and the HHS 405(d) Health Industry Cybersecurity Practices (HICP).
- Recognize current and pending rulemakings affecting HIPAA Security (December 2024 NPRM), reproductive health privacy, and Section 1557 nondiscrimination.
- Distinguish HIPAA scope from PCI DSS scope when healthcare organizations process card payments.

0.35 HIPAA: The Core Framework

The Health Insurance Portability and Accountability Act of 1996, as expanded by the HITECH Act (2009), the Omnibus Final Rule (2013), and the **HIPAA Privacy Rule on reproductive health information (NPRM 2023; Final Rule 2024)**, governs the handling of Protected Health Information (PHI) by covered entities and business associates. The reproductive health NPRM was published April 17, 2023 (88 FR 23506) and the corresponding Final Rule was published April 26, 2024 (89 FR 32976).

A **covered entity** is a health plan, healthcare clearinghouse, or health care provider that transmits any health information in electronic form in connection with a HIPAA transaction (45 CFR § 160.103). A **business associate** is a person or organization that performs certain functions or activities involving the use or disclosure of PHI on behalf of a covered entity.

The three principal rules:

Privacy Rule (45 CFR Part 160 and Part 164 Subparts A and E) — governs the use and disclosure of PHI. Core concepts:

- **Treatment, Payment, and Health Care Operations (TPO)** — PHI may be used and disclosed for these purposes without patient authorization.
- **Minimum necessary** — except for treatment, disclosures and uses must be limited to the minimum necessary to accomplish the purpose.
- **Individual rights** — access (right to inspect and obtain copy), amendment, accounting of disclosures, restriction request, confidential communications, notice of privacy practices.

Security Rule (45 CFR Part 160 and Part 164 Subparts A and C) — governs the confidentiality, integrity, and availability of electronic PHI (ePHI). The rule organizes safeguards into three categories with required and addressable specifications:

- **Administrative safeguards** — security management process (including the risk analysis), assigned security responsibility, workforce security, information access management, security awareness and training, security incident procedures, contingency plan, evaluation.
- **Physical safeguards** — facility access controls, workstation use and security, device and media controls.
- **Technical safeguards** — access control, audit controls, integrity, person or entity authentication, transmission security.

Breach Notification Rule (45 CFR Part 164 Subpart D) — requires covered entities to notify affected individuals, HHS, and (for breaches affecting 500 or more) the media of breaches of unsecured PHI. Individual notice must be sent without unreasonable delay and in no case later than 60 calendar days after discovery.

Breaches affecting 500 or more must be reported to HHS contemporaneously with individual notice; smaller breaches are reported annually within 60 days of the end of the calendar year.

"Secured" PHI is PHI rendered unusable through encryption that complies with NIST SP 800-111 (data at rest) or NIST SP 800-52 / SP 800-77 (data in motion). The Breach Notification Rule does not apply to secured PHI.

0.36 Pending Rulemaking: HIPAA Security Rule NPRM (December 2024)

In December 2024, HHS OCR published a Notice of Proposed Rulemaking that would substantially modernize the HIPAA Security Rule, which had not been comprehensively updated since 2013. As of early 2026, the rule remains an NPRM and has not been finalized; candidates should know its scope but not treat its provisions as currently enforceable. Key proposals include:

- **Mandatory multi-factor authentication (MFA)** for all access to ePHI (eliminating the existing "addressable" flexibility for authentication strengthening).
- **Mandatory encryption** of ePHI at rest and in transit (also moving from addressable to required).
- **Mandatory asset inventory and network map** — covered entities and business associates would be required to maintain a written inventory of technology assets and a network map illustrating ePHI flow.
- **Vulnerability scanning** at least every six months and **penetration testing** annually.
- **Mandatory written verification of business associate compliance** at least annually.
- **Mandatory incident response and contingency plan testing** with specific recovery time objectives.

OCR has signaled these provisions would have a 180-day compliance window after a final rule is published. Until the rule is finalized, the 2013-vintage Security Rule remains the enforceable baseline.

0.37 Risk Analysis and Risk Management

The **Security Management Process** standard (45 CFR § 164.308(a)(1)) requires every covered entity and business associate to:

1. Conduct an accurate and thorough **risk analysis** of vulnerabilities to the confidentiality, integrity, and availability of ePHI.
2. Implement **risk management** measures sufficient to reduce risks and vulnerabilities to a reasonable and appropriate level.
3. Apply **sanctions** to workforce members who violate policy.
4. Conduct **information system activity review** (audit log review).

The risk analysis is the most-cited deficiency in HHS Office for Civil Rights settlement actions. CAHIMS candidates should know that there is no required methodology, but NIST SP 800-30 Rev. 1 (Guide for Conducting Risk Assessments) and HHS's **Security Risk Assessment Tool (SRA Tool) v3.4** (updated 2024) are the most widely used references. NIST SP 800-66 Rev. 2 (February 2024) is the current implementation guide for the HIPAA Security Rule.

0.38 HHS 405(d) HICP

Section 405(d) of the Cybersecurity Act of 2015 directed HHS to develop voluntary cybersecurity practices for the health sector. The result is **Health Industry Cybersecurity Practices (HICP)** with editions tailored to small, medium, and large organizations. The 2023 update identifies five threats and ten practices:

Five threats: email phishing, ransomware, loss or theft of equipment/data, accidental or intentional data loss by insiders, attacks against connected medical devices.

Ten practices: email protection, endpoint protection, access management, data protection and loss prevention, asset management, network management, vulnerability management, incident response, medical device security, cybersecurity oversight and governance.

Under the **HITECH Act amendment of 2021** (Public Law 116-321), OCR must consider an organization's adoption of "recognized security practices" (including 405(d) HICP and the NIST Cybersecurity Framework) when determining fines and other remedies for HIPAA Security Rule violations.

0.39 Ransomware and Incident Response

Ransomware is the single most consequential cybersecurity threat to healthcare. The HHS HC3 sector report (2024) identified more than 250 distinct ransomware incidents affecting U.S. healthcare organizations in 2023. The 2024 Change Healthcare incident, attributed to ALPHV/BlackCat, disrupted billing and claims processing for weeks and exposed the records of an estimated 100 million individuals.

OCR's 2016 guidance clarifies that **ransomware on a system containing ePHI is presumptively a breach** unless the covered entity can demonstrate through a four-factor analysis a low probability that PHI was compromised. The four factors (45 CFR § 164.402):

1. Nature and extent of PHI involved.
2. Unauthorized person who used or received the PHI.
3. Whether PHI was actually acquired or viewed.
4. Extent to which the risk has been mitigated.

Standard ransomware controls include: phishing-resistant MFA (FIDO2 or hardware tokens) for privileged access, endpoint detection and response (EDR), email gateway protections, network segmentation (especially of medical-device VLANs), immutable backups stored off-network, and a tested incident response plan.

0.40 Identity and Access Management

The Security Rule's **Information Access Management** standard requires policies that authorize access to ePHI based on the user's role. **Role-Based Access Control (RBAC)** is the most common implementation. Many EHRs add **break-the-glass** controls that permit override for emergency access with mandatory audit logging.

Authentication standards in healthcare reference NIST SP 800-63-3 (Digital Identity Guidelines, with revisions through 800-63-4 expected). Common practices:

- **Multi-factor authentication (MFA)** for remote access, privileged accounts, and any internet-facing system. As noted above, the December 2024 HIPAA Security Rule NPRM proposes to make MFA an explicit, required safeguard for ePHI access; as of early 2026 this remains a proposed rule, and the existing Security Rule treats authentication strengthening as an addressable specification.
- **DEA EPCS (Electronic Prescribing of Controlled Substances)** — requires two-factor authentication using a token plus a knowledge factor (or biometric). The hardware token must meet **FIPS 140-2 Level 1 (or higher), as cited in 21 CFR 1311.115** (transitioning to FIPS 140-3 as NIST validations migrate; NIST retired FIPS 140-2 in 2022 but DEA has not formally updated 21 CFR 1311 to cite FIPS 140-3).
- **Single Sign-On (SSO)** via SAML 2.0 or OIDC to reduce password proliferation.

0.41 and Patient Care Decision Support Tools

The HHS **Section 1557 Final Rule** (signed April 26, 2024; published in the Federal Register May 6, 2024) prohibits discrimination on the basis of race, color, national origin, sex (including pregnancy, sexual orientation, and gender identity), age, or disability in federally funded health programs and activities. The rule establishes phased compliance dates:

- **July 5, 2024** — general effective date for most provisions.
- **May 1, 2025** — compliance date for the nondiscrimination provisions specific to **patient care decision support tools** at **45 CFR 92.210**, which require covered entities to identify uses of patient care decision support tools (including AI/ML and rule-based CDS) that employ input variables or factors measuring race, color, national origin, sex, age, or disability, and to make reasonable efforts to mitigate the risk of discrimination from such tools.
- **Various 2025–2026 dates** — for translated notices, accessibility of digital content, and other operational provisions.

The May 1, 2025 patient-care-decision-support-tool compliance date is the highest-yield Section 1557 fact for the 2026 exam.

0.42 PCI DSS Scope for Healthcare Organizations

Although HIPAA dominates healthcare information security discussions, healthcare organizations that **accept, process, store, or transmit cardholder data** for payment are subject to **PCI DSS (Payment Card Industry Data Security Standard)**, currently at version 4.0.1 (released June 2024, with version 4.0 fully effective March 31, 2025).

PCI DSS scope is **separate from HIPAA scope:**

- **HIPAA** governs PHI; PCI DSS governs cardholder data (primary account number, cardholder name, expiration date, service code, and sensitive authentication data).
- A hospital that takes patient copays via credit card is a PCI DSS merchant; the payment terminal, network segments handling card data, and any system that stores it (often the revenue cycle system or a third-party payment processor) are in PCI DSS scope.
- Network segmentation that isolates the cardholder data environment (CDE) from the broader hospital network typically reduces PCI DSS scope.
- A breach involving card data triggers PCI DSS reporting obligations (to acquiring banks and card brands) that are **separate from and additional to** any HIPAA Breach Notification Rule obligations if PHI was also involved.

PCI DSS and HIPAA are commonly confused on the exam; remember that PCI is contractual (enforced by acquiring banks and card brands), while HIPAA is regulatory (enforced by OCR).

> **Exam Tip**
>
> Ransomware that touches ePHI is *presumed* a breach. The four-factor analysis can rebut the presumption, but the default is to notify.

> **Exam Tip**
>
> Breach notification must be sent without unreasonable delay and no later than **60 calendar days** from discovery. Breaches affecting 500+ also require contemporaneous HHS and media notification.

> **Exam Tip**
>
> When a stem asks about "addressable" specifications under the Security Rule, remember that "addressable" does not mean optional — it means the organization must implement, document an alternative, or document why neither is reasonable and appropriate.

> **Exam Tip**
>
> For DEA EPCS, the regulation at 21 CFR 1311.115 still cites **FIPS 140-2 Level 1**, not 140-3. NIST retired 140-2 in 2022 but DEA has not formally updated the regulation. Answer with the regulation's text.

> **Exam Tip**
>
> When a stem mentions credit card payments at a hospital, think **PCI DSS**, not HIPAA — they are distinct and parallel obligations.

> **Key Concept**
>
> HIPAA's three core rules — Privacy, Security, Breach Notification — apply differently: Privacy covers all PHI, Security covers ePHI only, Breach Notification applies to unsecured PHI.

> **Key Concept**
>
> The Security Management Process requires a thorough risk analysis followed by documented risk management; absence of a current risk analysis is the most frequently cited HIPAA Security Rule deficiency.

Key Concept

"Recognized security practices" (405(d) HICP, NIST CSF) reduce OCR enforcement penalties if adopted, demonstrated, and maintained for the prior 12 months.

Key Concept

The December 2024 HIPAA Security NPRM would codify MFA, encryption, asset inventory, vulnerability scanning, and incident response testing as required safeguards — but it is an NPRM, not yet final.

0.43 Chapter 5 Review Questions

Q1. A hospital's EHR is encrypted with the vendor's FIPS 140-3 validated module. An employee laptop containing PHI is stolen. The laptop's drive was encrypted using BitLocker meeting NIST SP 800-111. Under the HIPAA Breach Notification Rule, the hospital must:
A) Notify all affected individuals within 60 days.
B) Notify OCR but not individuals.
C) Document the incident; notification is not required because the PHI was secured.
D) Pay a civil monetary penalty automatically.

Answer: C — Properly encrypted PHI is "secured" and is excepted from the Breach Notification Rule. The organization should still document the incident and reassess controls.

Q2. Which HIPAA standard requires that uses and disclosures of PHI be limited to what is needed to accomplish the purpose — except for treatment?
A) Privacy Rule "minimum necessary" standard
B) Security Rule "least privilege" standard
C) Breach Notification Rule "harm threshold"
D) HITECH Act "right of access"

Answer: A — The minimum necessary standard (45 CFR § 164.502(b)) applies to uses, disclosures, and requests other than for treatment.

Q3. A health system's IT director wants to invoke the "recognized security practices" mitigation if OCR investigates a future HIPAA Security Rule incident. Which framework is explicitly identified by statute as a recognized security practice?
A) ISO 27001
B) The HHS 405(d) HICP
C) PCI DSS 4.0
D) COBIT 2019

Answer: B — The 2021 amendment to HITECH (Public Law 116-321) names the HHS 405(d) practices and the NIST Cybersecurity Framework as recognized security practices.

Q4. A pharmacist must electronically prescribe a Schedule II controlled substance. Which authentication standard governs the cryptographic module used for the hardware token factor?
A) FIPS 140-3 Level 2 as required by 21 CFR Part 11
B) FIPS 140-2 Level 1 (or higher) as required by 21 CFR Part 1311
C) HIPAA Security Rule Person or Entity Authentication only
D) FIDO2 with platform authenticator only

Answer: B — DEA's EPCS rules (21 CFR Part 1311, including § 1311.115) require two-factor authentication with one factor on a hardware device meeting FIPS 140-2 Level 1 or higher. The DEA has not yet formally updated the CFR citation to FIPS 140-3.

Q5. A ransomware attack encrypts the imaging server's local storage; the EHR remains operational. Within how many calendar days, in the absence of a successful low-probability-of-compromise analysis, must individual notice be sent?
A) 30
B) 45
C) 60
D) 90

Answer: C — The HIPAA Breach Notification Rule requires individual notice without unreasonable delay and in no case later than 60 calendar days from discovery.

Healthcare Administration, Leadership, and Management

Approximate Exam Weight: 15%

0.44 Learning Objectives

After completing this chapter, the candidate will be able to:

- Identify organizational structures common to health systems (functional, matrix, service-line) and the IT governance bodies that operate within them.
- Apply project management fundamentals from PMBOK 7 and PRINCE2 to health-IT initiatives.
- Develop and defend IT budgets (operating, capital, total cost of ownership) for system investments.
- Lead change management efforts using established frameworks (Kotter, ADKAR, Prosci).
- Recognize FDA regulatory frameworks for AI/ML-enabled Software as a Medical Device, including Predetermined Change Control Plans (PCCP).

0.45 Health System Organizational Structures

Most U.S. hospitals and health systems exhibit a hybrid functional/matrix structure with a service-line overlay. The senior leadership team typically includes a CEO, COO, CFO, CMO, CNO, and CIO. Health IT–specific senior roles have grown:

- **Chief Medical Information Officer (CMIO)** — physician informaticist representing clinical interests in technology decisions.
- **Chief Nursing Information Officer (CNIO)** — counterpart for nursing.
- **Chief Information Security Officer (CISO)** — accountable for cybersecurity; reports to the CIO, COO, or directly to the CEO depending on organization.
- **Chief Digital Officer (CDO)** — oversees patient-facing digital experience, often distinct from the CIO role.
- **Chief Data Officer / Chief Analytics Officer** — accountable for data governance, analytics platforms, and AI/ML deployment.

The principal **IT governance bodies** typically include:

- **IT Steering Committee** — executive-level prioritization of major investments.
- **Clinical Informatics Council** — clinically led optimization governance.
- **Change Advisory Board (CAB)** — production change approval.
- **Data Governance Committee** — definitions, stewardship, and quality.
- **AI Governance Committee** (emerging) — review of clinical and administrative AI models before deployment, often using a framework derived from the **NIST AI Risk Management Framework (AI RMF 1.0, January 2023)** and the algorithmic discrimination provisions of the **HHS Section 1557 Final Rule at 45 CFR 92.210** (compliance date May 1, 2025).

0.46 Project Management Fundamentals

CAHIMS draws on **PMBOK 7** (Project Management Institute, published 2021) and to a lesser extent **PRINCE2 7** (released 2023 in the U.K.). PMBOK 7 reframes the earlier process-group view into eight **Project Performance Domains**: Stakeholders, Team, Development Approach and Life Cycle, Planning, Project Work, Delivery, Measurement, and Uncertainty. Candidates should know the names and intent but rarely need deeper detail.

The traditional **process groups** still appear in practice and on the exam:

1. **Initiating** — charter, identify stakeholders.
2. **Planning** — scope, schedule, cost, quality, resource, communications, risk, procurement, stakeholder engagement plans.

3. **Executing** — perform the work.
4. **Monitoring and Controlling** — track variance, manage change requests.
5. **Closing** — formal acceptance and lessons learned.

Specific tools and concepts to know:

- **Work Breakdown Structure (WBS)** — hierarchical decomposition of the project into deliverables.
- **Critical Path** — the longest sequence of dependent activities determining minimum project duration.
- **Earned Value Management (EVM)** — uses Planned Value (PV), Earned Value (EV), and Actual Cost (AC) to derive Cost Variance (CV = EV − AC), Schedule Variance (SV = EV − PV), Cost Performance Index (CPI = EV / AC), and Schedule Performance Index (SPI = EV / PV).
- **Risk register** — captures risks with probability, impact, owner, and response strategy (avoid, transfer, mitigate, accept).
- **Stakeholder register and engagement matrix** — categorizes stakeholders by power, interest, influence, and current vs. desired engagement.

0.47 IT Financial Management

CAHIMS expects literacy in two budget types and TCO:

Operating budget (OpEx) — recurring annual costs: salaries, software maintenance, support contracts, telecom, cloud subscriptions, training. OpEx is funded out of current revenue.

Capital budget (CapEx) — major investments depreciated over multiple years: hardware purchases, software licenses (when capitalized), construction. CapEx requires board approval at most health systems above a threshold (commonly $250K to $1M).

Cloud has shifted CapEx to OpEx — a SaaS EHR is OpEx; a customer-owned EHR is largely CapEx with OpEx maintenance. Finance committees increasingly demand TCO over five to seven years rather than year-one budget alone.

Common financial metrics:

- **Return on Investment (ROI)** = (Net Benefit / Cost) × 100%.
- **Net Present Value (NPV)** = discounted future cash flows minus initial investment.
- **Payback period** = time to recover the investment from net cash inflows.
- **Internal Rate of Return (IRR)** = the discount rate at which NPV = 0.

For health-IT investments, benefits include both **hard dollars** (denial reduction, length of stay reduction, FTE avoidance) and **soft dollars** (clinician satisfaction, regulatory protection, brand). Defensible ROI cases quantify the hard dollars and qualify the soft dollars.

0.48 Change Management Frameworks

System implementations fail more often from change management gaps than from technology gaps. CAHIMS tests recognition of major frameworks:

Kotter's 8-Step Model (John Kotter, *Leading Change*, 1996, refreshed 2014): create urgency, build a guiding coalition, form strategic vision, enlist a volunteer army, enable action by removing barriers, generate short-term wins, sustain acceleration, institute change.

ADKAR (Prosci): Awareness, Desire, Knowledge, Ability, Reinforcement. Individual-level model that complements organization-level frameworks.

Lewin's three-stage model: unfreeze, change, refreeze. The original model; still referenced as a conceptual anchor.

Bridges' Transitions Model: ending, neutral zone, new beginning. Emphasizes the psychological transition that follows external change.

In implementation governance, the practical change management plan includes a stakeholder analysis, communication plan (often with cadence and channel matrix), training plan, sponsorship plan, resistance management plan, and reinforcement plan.

0.49 FDA Regulation of AI/ML Software as a Medical Device

The FDA regulates software intended for diagnosis, treatment, prevention, cure, or mitigation of disease — including AI/ML algorithms — as **Software as a Medical Device (SaMD)** under the 21st Century Cures Act framework. Traditional FDA clearance pathways (510(k), De Novo, PMA) require sponsors to submit a new application for each significant modification to a cleared device, an approach that does not match the iterative retraining cycle of machine-learning models.

The FDA's **Predetermined Change Control Plan (PCCP)** framework, with final guidance issued in December 2024 (*Marketing Submission Recommendations for a Predetermined Change Control Plan for Artificial Intelligence/-Machine Learning (AI/ML)-Enabled Device Software Functions*), allows sponsors to pre-specify and obtain FDA authorization for planned modifications to an AI/ML device before those modifications are implemented. A PCCP includes:

- A **description of modifications** the sponsor intends to make.
- A **modification protocol** describing the methods used to develop, validate, and implement the modifications.
- An **impact assessment** evaluating the benefits and risks of the planned modifications.

Once a PCCP is authorized as part of an initial submission, the sponsor may implement the pre-specified modifications without filing a new 510(k) or supplemental PMA, provided the changes remain within the PCCP. The framework is especially relevant to continuously learning clinical algorithms used in radiology, cardiology, pathology, and ICU early-warning systems.

0.50 Leadership and Ethical Frameworks

Beyond frameworks, CAHIMS expects awareness of the leadership competencies the **AONL (American Organization for Nursing Leadership)** and **ACHE (American College of Healthcare Executives)** have published. The ACHE Competencies Assessment Tool groups competencies into communication and relationship management, leadership, professionalism, knowledge of the healthcare environment, and business knowledge and skills.

CAHIMS also touches on **ethical use of data and AI**. The HHS Section 1557 Final Rule (signed April 26, 2024; published May 6, 2024; patient-care-decision-support-tool compliance date May 1, 2025) prohibits discrimination by covered entities in their use of patient care decision support tools — including algorithms — that take into account race, color, national origin, sex, age, or disability. Health systems are obligated under 45 CFR 92.210 to identify whether each clinical decision support algorithm in use considers a protected characteristic and to make reasonable efforts to mitigate any resulting discrimination.

> **Exam Tip**
>
> EVM formulas reliably appear on CAHIMS: CV = EV − AC; SV = EV − PV; CPI = EV / AC; SPI = EV / PV. CPI and SPI > 1 are favorable.

> **Exam Tip**
>
> When a stem mentions "individual-level" change management, the answer is ADKAR. When it mentions "organization-level" or eight steps, the answer is Kotter.

> **Exam Tip**
>
> Section 1557 (2024 Final Rule) extends nondiscrimination obligations to algorithmic decision support at 45 CFR 92.210; the compliance date for that specific provision is **May 1, 2025.**

> **Exam Tip**
>
> When a question describes an AI/ML algorithm that will be retrained on new data after FDA clearance, think **Predetermined Change Control Plan (PCCP)** — FDA's December 2024 final guidance is the canonical reference.

> **Key Concept**

> Health IT governance distributes decision rights across an executive steering committee, a clinical informatics council, a change advisory board, a data governance committee, and (increasingly) an AI governance committee.

> **Key Concept**
> Capital vs. operating budgets, and the OpEx shift driven by SaaS and cloud, shape every business case; TCO is the proper lens for multi-year decisions.

> **Key Concept**
> Change management is not a communication plan. It is an integrated discipline that combines sponsorship, training, resistance management, and reinforcement — and ADKAR, Kotter, Lewin, and Bridges are the dominant frameworks.

0.51 Chapter 6 Review Questions

Q1. A project has a Planned Value of $500,000, Earned Value of $450,000, and Actual Cost of $480,000 through month five. What is the Cost Performance Index?

A) 0.90
B) 0.94
C) 0.96
D) 1.07

Answer: B — CPI = EV / AC = 450,000 / 480,000 = 0.9375, which rounds to 0.94. A CPI below 1.0 indicates the project is over budget.

Q2. A CIO wants to deploy a vendor-supplied sepsis prediction model in the EHR. Section 1557 (2024 Final Rule) at 45 CFR 92.210 requires the organization to:

A) Use the model only if FDA cleared.
B) Identify whether the model considers race, color, national origin, sex, age, or disability and make reasonable efforts to mitigate discrimination.
C) Obtain individual patient consent before each model run.
D) Disclose the model's source code to all clinical users.

Answer: B — Section 1557 (2024) at 45 CFR 92.210 requires identification and reasonable mitigation of potential discrimination when patient care decision support tools take into account protected characteristics. The compliance date for this provision is May 1, 2025.

Q3. Which change management framework is most often described as an individual-level model emphasizing Awareness, Desire, Knowledge, Ability, and Reinforcement?

A) Kotter's 8-Step Model
B) ADKAR
C) Lewin's three-stage model
D) Bridges' Transitions Model

Answer: B — ADKAR, developed by Prosci, is the canonical individual-level change framework.

Q4. A health system is selecting between purchasing an on-premises EHR (large CapEx with smaller OpEx) and subscribing to a SaaS EHR (no CapEx, larger OpEx). Which evaluation lens best supports the decision?

A) Year-one budget comparison
B) Five- to seven-year Total Cost of Ownership analysis
C) Single-year ROI
D) Payback period only

Answer: B — Multi-year TCO accounts for the OpEx/CapEx tradeoff, support, refresh cycles, and integration costs that distort year-one comparisons.

Q5. Which governance body is typically responsible for reviewing and approving proposed changes to the production EHR before deployment?

A) IT Steering Committee
B) Clinical Informatics Council
C) Change Advisory Board (CAB)

D) Data Governance Committee

Answer: C — The CAB reviews change requests, assesses risk and scheduling conflicts, and approves production changes.

0.52 Practice Exam

The following 50 multiple-choice questions cover all six domains in roughly the same proportions as the live exam. Allocate approximately one hour. After scoring, return to the chapter for any domain in which you missed more than two questions.

Q1. Under the 21st Century Cures Act Information Blocking Rule, civil monetary penalties may be assessed against developers of certified health IT, HIEs, and HINs of up to:

A) $100,000 per violation
B) $250,000 per violation
C) $1,000,000 per violation
D) $5,000,000 per violation

Answer: C — OIG's 2023 final rule established CMP penalties up to $1 million per violation for developers, HIEs, and HINs that engage in information blocking.

Q2. Which interoperability standard is required for the (g)(10) Standardized API certification criterion?

A) HL7 v2.5.1
B) HL7 CDA R2
C) HL7 FHIR R4 with US Core
D) HL7 FHIR R5

Answer: C — FHIR R4 with US Core IG and SMART App Launch is the (g)(10) requirement.

Q3. Within how many calendar days must individual notification of an unsecured-PHI breach be sent?

A) 30
B) 45
C) 60
D) 90

Answer: C — The Breach Notification Rule requires individual notice no later than 60 calendar days from discovery.

Q4. A nurse charts an allergy in the EHR; the system updates the patient's record and propagates the alert to all order entry screens. Which property of the data is preserved by the propagation?

A) Confidentiality
B) Integrity
C) Availability
D) Non-repudiation

Answer: B — Integrity is the property that data remains accurate and consistent across systems.

Q5. Which CMS payment program rewards or penalizes hospitals based on quality and efficiency measures, redistributing about 2% of IPPS payments?

A) Hospital Readmissions Reduction Program
B) Hospital-Acquired Condition Reduction Program
C) Hospital Value-Based Purchasing Program
D) MIPS

Answer: C — Hospital VBP redistributes approximately 2% of IPPS payments.

Q6. A practice receives an X12 271 transaction. This indicates:

A) A claim has been submitted.
B) Eligibility verification has been returned.
C) Remittance advice has been received.
D) Prior authorization has been granted.

Answer: B — X12 271 is the eligibility verification response paired with the 270 request.

Q7. The principal terminology for clinical concepts (problems, findings) in USCDI is:

A) ICD-10-CM
B) SNOMED CT
C) CPT

D) HCPCS

Answer: B — SNOMED CT is the USCDI-required terminology for problems and findings.

Q8. Which integration engine pattern decouples sending and receiving systems so that the addition of a new downstream consumer does not require changes upstream?

A) Direct point-to-point
B) Hub-and-spoke with publish/subscribe topics
C) FTP file drops
D) Email forwarding

Answer: B — Hub-and-spoke publish/subscribe is the canonical decoupling pattern.

Q9. A health system has chosen a phased rollout across six hospitals, six weeks apart. The first hospital go-live experiences unexpected pharmacy interface failures. The appropriate response is to:

A) Cancel all subsequent waves.
B) Convene incident management to restore service while problem management investigates root cause.
C) Roll back the EHR.
D) Switch to a big bang for the remaining sites.

Answer: B — Incident management restores service; problem management investigates root cause. Decisions about subsequent waves should follow root-cause analysis.

Q10. Which document records the impact of risks to a project along with planned responses?

A) Stakeholder register
B) Issue log
C) Risk register
D) Change log

Answer: C — A risk register captures risks with probability, impact, and response strategy.

Q11. The HIPAA Security Rule organizes safeguards into administrative, physical, and technical categories. Workstation security is a:

A) Administrative safeguard
B) Physical safeguard
C) Technical safeguard
D) Policy safeguard

Answer: B — Workstation security and workstation use are physical safeguards under 45 CFR § 164.310.

Q12. A vendor processes PHI on behalf of a covered entity. The vendor stores the PHI exclusively in encrypted form and holds no decryption keys. Under HIPAA, the vendor is:

A) Not a business associate because it cannot read the PHI.
B) A business associate and must execute a BAA.
C) A covered entity.
D) A clearinghouse.

Answer: B — OCR's 2016 cloud guidance is explicit that ciphertext-only providers are still business associates and require BAAs.

Q13. A clinical decision support rule fires whenever a serum potassium of >5.5 mEq/L is resulted and stops the next nephrotoxic drug order until a clinician acknowledges. Which type of CDS is this?

A) Order-entry alert
B) Documentation template
C) Order set
D) Patient education

Answer: A — This is an order-entry alert tied to a structured result.

Q14. The U.S. Core Data for Interoperability (USCDI) v4 includes which of the following data classes?

A) Wallet identifiers
B) Health Insurance Information
C) Genome sequencing
D) Banking transactions

Answer: B — USCDI v4 (July 2023) added Health Insurance Information among other data classes.

Q15. A six-hospital rollout that lights up all modules at every site on the same day is best described as:

A) Phased
B) Big bang
C) Parallel

D) Pilot

Answer: B — Same-day, all-modules, all-sites is a big bang.

Q16. A provider's MIPS score in 2026 is built from four categories with which weighting?

A) Quality 50%, Cost 10%, IA 10%, PI 30%
B) Quality 30%, Cost 30%, IA 15%, PI 25%
C) Quality 25%, Cost 25%, IA 25%, PI 25%
D) Quality 40%, Cost 20%, IA 20%, PI 20%

Answer: B — For 2026, Quality 30%, Cost 30%, Improvement Activities 15%, Promoting Interoperability 25%.

Q17. The NIST publication that provides guidance on media sanitization is:

A) NIST SP 800-30 Rev. 1
B) NIST SP 800-53 Rev. 5
C) NIST SP 800-66 Rev. 2
D) NIST SP 800-88 Rev. 1

Answer: D — NIST SP 800-88 Rev. 1 covers Clear, Purge, and Destroy categories.

Q18. The HHS publication providing voluntary cybersecurity practices for health sector organizations is:

A) HHS HC3 advisory
B) HHS 405(d) HICP
C) HHS Notice of Privacy Practices
D) HHS Office of Inspector General Workplan

Answer: B — HICP is the 405(d) deliverable, with tailored editions for small, medium, and large organizations.

Q19. ePCR (Electronic Patient Care Reporting) systems are most associated with which care setting?

A) Inpatient acute care
B) Pre-hospital EMS
C) Outpatient behavioral health
D) Home health

Answer: B — ePCR is the standard documentation format for pre-hospital emergency medical services.

Q20. A clinic uses athenaOne, hosted by athenahealth in athenahealth's data centers, billed monthly per provider. Which cloud service model best describes this?

A) IaaS
B) PaaS
C) SaaS
D) FaaS

Answer: C — A fully managed application delivered over the web with per-provider subscription billing is SaaS.

Q21. The HIPAA Privacy Rule's **Final Rule** on reproductive health information was published by HHS OCR in:

A) 2020
B) 2022
C) 2023
D) 2024

Answer: D — HHS OCR published the Final Rule on reproductive health information on April 26, 2024 (89 FR 32976). The corresponding Notice of Proposed Rulemaking was published earlier, on April 17, 2023 (88 FR 23506).

Q22. A clinical informaticist diagrams the OR turnover process to identify steps that do not add value. Which Lean technique is in use?

A) PDCA cycle
B) Value Stream Map
C) 5 Whys
D) Fishbone diagram

Answer: B — VSM distinguishes value-added from non-value-added time.

Q23. A NIST framework that provides a common language for managing cybersecurity risk is:

A) NIST SP 800-30
B) NIST Cybersecurity Framework (CSF) 2.0
C) NIST SP 800-88
D) NIST SP 800-66

Answer: B — NIST CSF 2.0 (released February 2024) provides the common language and Govern, Identify, Protect, Detect, Respond, Recover functions.

Q24. Which transaction is used to request prior authorization under HIPAA's electronic transaction standards?

A) X12 270
B) X12 276
C) X12 278
D) X12 835

Answer: C — X12 278 is the services review (prior authorization) transaction.

Q25. A breach affecting 500 individuals in a single state must be reported to which entities at the time of individual notification?

A) HHS only
B) HHS and prominent media outlets
C) State Attorney General only
D) FBI and HHS

Answer: B — Breaches affecting 500+ require contemporaneous notice to HHS and prominent media outlets serving the affected jurisdiction.

Q26. A health system board is asked to approve $12 million for a new EHR. The investment requires depreciation over seven years. This is a:

A) Operating budget request
B) Capital budget request
C) Discretionary expense
D) Bridge financing

Answer: B — A multi-year depreciable asset request is a capital budget request.

Q27. Which ITIL practice ensures that an accurate inventory of components and relationships supports change impact analysis?

A) Incident management
B) Change management
C) Configuration management
D) Release management

Answer: C — Configuration management maintains the CMDB.

Q28. Which framework is most often referenced for individual-level change adoption?

A) Kotter
B) ADKAR
C) Lewin
D) Bridges

Answer: B — ADKAR is the individual-level framework.

Q29. The principal regulation governing electronic prescribing of controlled substances is:

A) 45 CFR Part 164
B) 21 CFR Part 1311
C) 42 CFR Part 2
D) 21 CFR Part 11

Answer: B — DEA's EPCS rules are at 21 CFR Part 1311.

Q30. A clinical decision support intervention that requires clinicians to enter a reason before overriding is best described as a:

A) Hard stop
B) Soft alert with reason capture
C) Order set
D) Patient education prompt

Answer: B — A soft alert with mandatory reason capture allows override with documentation; a hard stop would not allow override.

Q31. Patient-reported outcomes captured through digital surveys are most commonly stored in:

A) The PACS
B) The EHR via FHIR Questionnaire/QuestionnaireResponse
C) The HL7 v2 ORM message
D) The X12 837 claim

Answer: B — FHIR Questionnaire and QuestionnaireResponse resources are the standard for capturing PROs.

Q32. Substance use disorder records held by federally assisted programs are governed by which regulation in addition to HIPAA?

A) 42 CFR Part 2
B) 45 CFR Part 160
C) 21 CFR Part 11
D) 29 CFR Part 1910

Answer: A — 42 CFR Part 2 imposes a stricter consent standard for SUD records.

Q33. When did the first QHINs become operational under TEFCA?

A) 2018
B) 2020
C) 2023
D) 2025

Answer: C — The TEFCA Common Agreement v1.0 was published January 2022; the first five QHINs (eHealth Exchange, Epic Nexus, Health Gorilla, KONZA, and MedAllies) were designated and became operational in December 2023.

Q34. Which OASIS edition is in effect for home health assessment as of January 1, 2025?

A) OASIS-C
B) OASIS-D1
C) OASIS-E
D) OASIS-E1

Answer: D — OASIS-E1 took effect January 1, 2025.

Q35. A network of regional integrated delivery systems shares clinical data using IHE XDS.b document repository and registry profiles. This pattern is most consistent with:

A) HL7 v2 over MLLP
B) Direct Secure Messaging
C) Query-based health information exchange
D) FHIR Subscription

Answer: C — XDS.b underpins query-based document exchange used by HIEs.

Q36. Which performance metric measures the ratio of value earned to actual cost?

A) Schedule Performance Index
B) Cost Performance Index
C) Schedule Variance
D) Cost Variance

Answer: B — CPI = EV / AC.

Q37. A vendor's SLA specifies a 15-minute response and a 4-hour restoration target for outages of the production EHR. This level is most consistent with:

A) Severity 1
B) Severity 2
C) Severity 3
D) Severity 4

Answer: A — Sev 1 typically denotes system down with patient safety risk and the most aggressive response/restoration targets.

Q38. HIPAA's "addressable" specification means:

A) Optional and may be skipped.
B) Required, but implementation method may be alternate if documented as reasonable and appropriate.
C) Required, with no flexibility.
D) Only applies to large organizations.

Answer: B — Addressable does not mean optional; the organization must implement, document an alternative, or document that neither is reasonable and appropriate.

Q39. A health system's CISO wants to defend the organization's cybersecurity posture during an OCR investigation by demonstrating recognized security practices for the past 12 months. Which framework qualifies?

A) NIST CSF 2.0
B) ISO 9001
C) ITIL 4

D) PMBOK 7

Answer: A — NIST CSF and HHS 405(d) HICP are statutorily recognized security practices.

Q40. Which type of testing involves end clinical users executing real-world scenarios on the configured system before go-live?

A) Unit testing
B) Integration testing
C) User acceptance testing
D) Regression testing

Answer: C — UAT is end-user, scenario-based testing before formal acceptance.

Q41. A revenue cycle director wants to reduce denials by integrating eligibility verification with scheduling. Which X12 transaction must the EHR send to verify eligibility before the appointment?

A) X12 270
B) X12 276
C) X12 278
D) X12 837

Answer: A — X12 270 is the eligibility inquiry; 271 is the response.

Q42. A small ambulatory practice cannot afford a full disaster recovery site. The practice uses encrypted cloud backups with documented restore procedures tested annually. Under the HIPAA Security Rule, this is most consistent with which standard?

A) Risk analysis
B) Contingency plan
C) Access control
D) Audit controls

Answer: B — The Contingency Plan standard (164.308(a)(7)) requires data backup, disaster recovery, and emergency mode operation plans.

Q43. A patient-portal screen allowing a patient to download her medications and allergies via the FHIR US Core Patient access scope is enabled by:

A) The MyChart proprietary API
B) The (g)(10) Standardized API certification criterion
C) The X12 270 transaction
D) The DICOM C-STORE operation

Answer: B — The (g)(10) criterion mandates FHIR R4 patient access supported by US Core scopes and SMART App Launch.

Q44. Which ONC criterion underpins the C-CDA-based transitions of care document exchange?

A) § 170.315(a)(1)
B) § 170.315(b)(1)
C) § 170.315(d)(1)
D) § 170.315(g)(10)

Answer: B — § 170.315(b)(1) covers transitions of care.

Q45. A new AI-based clinical decision support model is to be deployed across 12 inpatient units. The most appropriate governance body to review the model before deployment is:

A) Change Advisory Board
B) AI Governance / Data & Analytics governance committee
C) Pharmacy and Therapeutics Committee
D) Infection Prevention Committee

Answer: B — AI / Data & Analytics governance is the body specifically formed to evaluate model risk, performance, and equity.

Q46. A telehealth visit with both audio and video using a HIPAA-compliant platform requires which technical safeguards?

A) Transmission security (encryption in transit) and authentication
B) Workstation security only
C) Audit controls only
D) Facility access controls only

Answer: A — Transmission security and person/entity authentication are the directly applicable technical safeguards.

Q47. A community hospital's CIO is choosing between a five-year contract for a Hosted EHR and a seven-year contract for an on-premises EHR. Which analysis would best inform the choice?

A) Year-one capital outlay only
B) TCO across seven years including transition costs
C) Vendor reference score only
D) RFP score only

Answer: B — TCO across the longer horizon captures both options' costs and avoids the year-one distortion.

Q48. A health system uses Slack to discuss patient cases. Without a BAA and HIPAA-compliant configuration, this practice:

A) Is acceptable as long as participants are credentialed.
B) Is a HIPAA violation because PHI is being disclosed to a business associate without a BAA and without minimum-necessary controls.
C) Is allowed under the treatment exception.
D) Is allowed if participants use private channels.

Answer: B — Disclosure of PHI to a business associate without a BAA and without minimum-necessary controls is a HIPAA violation.

Q49. The HHS Section 1557 Final Rule (2024) primarily addresses:

A) Mental health parity
B) Nondiscrimination in healthcare programs, including in patient care decision support tools
C) Surprise billing
D) Medicare Advantage marketing

Answer: B — The 2024 Section 1557 Final Rule extends nondiscrimination obligations to algorithmic decision support tools at 45 CFR 92.210, with a May 1, 2025 compliance date for that specific provision.

Q50. A CAHIMS candidate is asked which standard is appropriate for sharing imaging studies across organizations using a common metadata header and a defined transfer protocol. The candidate should answer:

A) HL7 v2
B) HL7 FHIR
C) DICOM with IHE XDS-I
D) X12 837I

Answer: C — DICOM defines imaging interchange; IHE XDS-I packages DICOM for cross-enterprise imaging exchange.

Exam Quick Reference

Exam mechanics. 115 items (100 scored, 15 unscored pilot). Two hours. Passing scaled score 70/100. Pearson VUE testing centers or OnVUE remote proctoring. No penalty for guessing.

Key federal references. - HIPAA Privacy Rule: 45 CFR Parts 160, 164 Subparts A, E. - HIPAA Privacy Rule — Reproductive Health Information: NPRM published April 17, 2023 (88 FR 23506); Final Rule published April 26, 2024 (89 FR 32976). - HIPAA Security Rule: 45 CFR Parts 160, 164 Subparts A, C. Modernization NPRM published December 2024 (proposes mandatory MFA, encryption, asset inventory, vulnerability scanning); not yet final as of early 2026. - HIPAA Breach Notification Rule: 45 CFR Part 164 Subpart D. - 42 CFR Part 2 — Substance Use Disorder records. - 21 CFR Part 1311 — DEA EPCS; cites FIPS 140-2 Level 1 for hardware tokens (transition to FIPS 140-3 pending). - 21st Century Cures Act, ONC Final Rule (Information Blocking), OIG CMP Final Rule (2023). - ONC HTI-1 Final Rule (December 2023) — Decision Support Interventions criterion at § 170.315(b)(11); USCDI v3 transition. - CMS Interoperability and Prior Authorization Final Rule (CMS-0057-F, January 2024) — Patient Access, Provider Access, Payer-to-Payer, and Prior Authorization APIs (effective 2026–2027). - ASTP/ONC HTI-2 Proposed Rule (2024) — public health interoperability, payer-provider FHIR exchange. - FDA Predetermined Change Control Plan final guidance (December 2024) — AI/ML SaMD modifications without new 510(k). - Section 1557 Final Rule — signed April 26, 2024; published May 6, 2024; general effective date July 5, 2024; algorithmic CDS nondiscrimination (45 CFR 92.210) compliance date **May 1, 2025.**

Interoperability standards. - HL7 v2 — messaging over MLLP. - HL7 CDA / C-CDA — XML clinical documents. - HL7 FHIR R4 — RESTful API; required for ONC (g)(10). - DICOM — imaging. - NCPDP SCRIPT — e-prescribing. - X12 270/271, 276/277, 278, 834, 835, 837 — administrative.

Terminologies. - ICD-10-CM (diagnoses), ICD-10-PCS (inpatient procedures). - CPT (outpatient procedures), HCPCS II (supplies, DME). - SNOMED CT (clinical concepts), LOINC (observations, maintained by Regenstrief Institute), RxNorm (drugs). - UCUM (units of measure, Regenstrief Institute), CVX/MVX, USCDI v4.

Key MIPS 2026 weights: Quality 30%, Cost 30%, IA 15%, PI 25%.

Breach notification timing: 60 calendar days individual; contemporaneous HHS and media for ≥500.

ITIL practices to remember: incident, problem, change, release, configuration, service request.

Earned Value formulas: CV=EV−AC; SV=EV−PV; CPI=EV/AC; SPI=EV/PV.

Change frameworks: Kotter (org-level, 8 steps), ADKAR (individual, 5 elements), Lewin (unfreeze/change/refreeze), Bridges (ending/neutral zone/new beginning).

Recognized security practices: NIST CSF 2.0, HHS 405(d) HICP — must be in place 12 months to be considered by OCR.

Cloud service models: IaaS (infrastructure), PaaS (platform), SaaS (software).

Cutover strategies: big bang, phased, parallel, pilot.

TEFCA: Trusted Exchange Framework and Common Agreement; QHINs are the on-ramps for nationwide network-of-networks exchange. First five QHINs designated December 2023; CommonWell designated February 2024; further additions through 2024–2025.

Distinguish HIPAA from PCI DSS: HIPAA governs PHI (regulatory, OCR-enforced); PCI DSS 4.0.1 governs cardholder data (contractual, card-brand-enforced). A hospital that accepts card payments is subject to both regimes, with separate scopes, controls, and breach-reporting obligations.

Joint Commission Sentinel Event Policy: patient safety events resulting in death, permanent harm, or severe temporary harm. Health-IT–related sentinel events (wrong-patient EHR errors, CDS failures, interface failures) require comprehensive systematic analysis and corrective action plan within 55 business days of reporting.

Exam Quick Reference

Glossary

ACO REACH — CMS Innovation Center accountable care model that replaced Direct Contracting in 2023.

Accreditation — formal recognition by a body (e.g., The Joint Commission) that an organization meets specified standards.

ADKAR — individual-level change management model (Awareness, Desire, Knowledge, Ability, Reinforcement).

ADT — Admission, Discharge, Transfer messaging in HL7 v2.

AI Governance Committee — emerging governance body that reviews AI models before clinical deployment.

API — Application Programming Interface; in healthcare, the dominant API standard is HL7 FHIR.

ASTP — Assistant Secretary for Technology Policy; 2024 rebrand of ONC's parent organization, continuing to administer the ONC Health IT Certification Program.

BAA — Business Associate Agreement; mandatory HIPAA contract between covered entity and business associate.

Big Bang — cutover strategy in which all modules go live at all locations simultaneously.

Business Associate — person or entity that performs functions involving the use or disclosure of PHI on behalf of a covered entity.

CAB — Change Advisory Board; governs production changes.

CAHIMS — Certified Associate in Healthcare Information and Management Systems.

Capital Budget (CapEx) — multi-year depreciable spending.

C-CDA — Consolidated Clinical Document Architecture; C-CDA R2.1 templates are widely used.

Certification (ONC) — ONC Health IT Certification Program qualifies health IT to specific § 170.315 criteria.

CMS — Centers for Medicare & Medicaid Services.

CMDB — Configuration Management Database.

CMS Interoperability and Prior Authorization Final Rule — CMS-0057-F (January 2024); requires impacted payers to implement Patient Access, Provider Access, Payer-to-Payer, and Prior Authorization APIs (effective 2026–2027).

Covered Entity — health plan, healthcare clearinghouse, or health care provider that transmits health information electronically in connection with a HIPAA transaction.

CPOE — Computerized Provider Order Entry.

CPT — Current Procedural Terminology (AMA); used for outpatient procedure billing.

DICOM — Digital Imaging and Communications in Medicine.

Direct Secure Messaging — Direct Trust-accredited SMTP-with-S/MIME exchange between HISPs.

DSI — Decision Support Intervention; certification criterion at § 170.315(b)(11) introduced by ONC HTI-1 Final Rule (December 2023). Predictive DSIs require source-attribute transparency.

EHR — Electronic Health Record.

EPCS — Electronic Prescribing of Controlled Substances; regulated under 21 CFR Part 1311; hardware token must meet FIPS 140-2 Level 1 per § 1311.115.

Earned Value Management (EVM) — project performance technique using PV, EV, AC and derived indices.

FHIR — Fast Healthcare Interoperability Resources; RESTful API standard.

FIPS 140-2 / 140-3 — NIST Federal Information Processing Standards for cryptographic modules. NIST retired FIPS 140-2 in 2022, but 21 CFR 1311.115 (DEA EPCS) still cites FIPS 140-2 Level 1.

HCPCS Level II — codes for supplies, DME, drugs; maintained by CMS.

HICP — Health Industry Cybersecurity Practices (HHS 405(d)).

HIE / HIN — Health Information Exchange / Health Information Network.

HIMSS — Healthcare Information and Management Systems Society; the credentialing body for CAHIMS and CPHIMS.

HIPAA — Health Insurance Portability and Accountability Act of 1996.

HITECH — Health Information Technology for Economic and Clinical Health Act (2009).

HTI-1 — ONC Final Rule (December 2023) introducing the DSI certification criterion and updating USCDI/US Core baselines on a phased schedule.

HTI-2 — ASTP/ONC Proposed Rule (2024) extending interoperability to public health and payer-provider FHIR exchange.

HL7 v2 — pipe-and-hat delimited messaging standard.
ICD-10-CM / PCS — diagnosis codes (CM) and inpatient procedure codes (PCS).
Incident — unplanned interruption to service; restored via incident management.
Information Blocking — practices likely to interfere with EHI access, exchange, or use, prohibited under the 21st Century Cures Act.
ITIL 4 — service management framework.
Joint Commission (TJC) — CMS-deemed hospital accreditor.
LOINC — Logical Observation Identifiers Names and Codes; maintained by the Regenstrief Institute.
MIPS — Merit-based Incentive Payment System.
MDS 3.0 — Minimum Data Set 3.0; SNF assessment.
NCPDP SCRIPT — e-prescribing standard.
NIST CSF — NIST Cybersecurity Framework; CSF 2.0 released February 2024.
NIST SP 800-30 / 800-66 / 800-88 — guides for risk assessment, HIPAA Security Rule implementation, and media sanitization respectively.
ONC — Office of the National Coordinator for Health Information Technology (administered by ASTP since 2024).
OASIS-E1 — Outcome and Assessment Information Set for home health; effective January 1, 2025.
Operating Budget (OpEx) — recurring annual operating expense.
PACS — Picture Archiving and Communication System.
PCCP — Predetermined Change Control Plan; FDA framework (final guidance December 2024) for pre-authorizing modifications to AI/ML-enabled SaMD.
PCI DSS — Payment Card Industry Data Security Standard (current version 4.0.1, June 2024). Governs cardholder data; separate from HIPAA. Applies to any healthcare organization that accepts, processes, stores, or transmits card payments.
PCMH — Patient-Centered Medical Home; NCQA recognition.
PHI — Protected Health Information.
Privacy Rule — HIPAA rule governing use and disclosure of PHI.
Problem Management — investigation of root cause across one or more incidents.
QHIN — Qualified Health Information Network under TEFCA.
Recognized Security Practices — NIST CSF and HHS 405(d) HICP, statutorily considered by OCR.
Regenstrief Institute — Indiana-based research organization that maintains LOINC and UCUM.
RFI / RFP — Request for Information / Request for Proposal.
RBAC — Role-Based Access Control.
RxNorm — NLM's normalized naming system for clinical drugs.
SaMD — Software as a Medical Device; FDA-regulated software intended for diagnosis, treatment, prevention, cure, or mitigation of disease.
Section 1557 — ACA nondiscrimination provision; 2024 final rule extends to algorithmic CDS at 45 CFR 92.210 (May 1, 2025 compliance date for that provision).
Sentinel Event — Joint Commission term for a patient safety event resulting in death, permanent harm, or severe temporary harm. Health-IT–related sentinel events include wrong-patient EHR errors, CDS failures, and interface failures with clinical consequence.
SLA — Service Level Agreement.
SMART App Launch — open standard layered on FHIR and OAuth 2.0 to launch authorized health apps.
SNOMED CT — Systematized Nomenclature of Medicine — Clinical Terms.
TCO — Total Cost of Ownership.
TEFCA — Trusted Exchange Framework and Common Agreement.
Terminology — coded vocabulary used in clinical or financial systems.
Three Lines of Defense — model: operations, oversight, internal audit.
Transitions of Care — handoffs of patient information across settings; supported by C-CDA and FHIR.
UCUM — Unified Code for Units of Measure; maintained by the Regenstrief Institute.
Unsecured PHI — PHI not rendered unusable through encryption or destruction per HHS guidance; subject to Breach Notification Rule.
USCDI — United States Core Data for Interoperability; v4 effective for 2026 certification; v3 referenced in HTI-1 phased compliance schedule.
Value-Based Care — care models that tie reimbursement to outcomes and total cost of care.

Vendor Risk Management — discipline of assessing and monitoring third-party risk.
WBS — Work Breakdown Structure.
Zero Trust — security model that assumes breach and verifies every session and device.

Study Schedule

.1 Four-Week Intensive Plan (15–20 hours per week)

Week 1 — Industry and Technology Environment - Day 1–2: Read Chapter 1; complete Chapter 1 review questions; review rationales. - Day 3–4: Read Chapter 2; build a flashcard deck of standards (HL7, FHIR, DICOM, X12) and the 2023–2024 federal rulemakings (HTI-1, CMS Interop/PA, HTI-2). - Day 5: Practice ten standards-identification questions; review missed items. - Day 6: Read first half of Chapter 3 (SDLC, workflow analysis). - Day 7: Light review; cumulative review questions from Chapters 1–2.

Week 2 — Systems Lifecycle and Implementation - Day 1: Read second half of Chapter 3; complete Chapter 3 questions. - Day 2–3: Read Chapter 4; build cutover-strategy and ITIL practice flashcards; review Joint Commission Sentinel Event Policy. - Day 4: Practice ten EVM and project management questions. - Day 5–6: Review weak areas; complete cumulative review of Chapters 1–4. - Day 7: Half practice exam (Q1–Q25); review every missed rationale.

Week 3 — Privacy, Security, and Administration - Day 1–2: Read Chapter 5; flashcards for HIPAA standards, NIST publications, breach timing, PCI DSS vs HIPAA scope, December 2024 Security NPRM provisions, and the FIPS 140-2 / 21 CFR 1311 EPCS citation. - Day 3–4: Read Chapter 6; flashcards for change frameworks, EVM formulas, governance bodies, FDA PCCP, and Section 1557 phased compliance dates. - Day 5: Practice fifteen privacy/security questions and ten administration questions. - Day 6: Cumulative review of weak domains. - Day 7: Half practice exam (Q26–Q50); score and triage.

Week 4 — Integration and Drilling - Day 1: Full 50-question practice exam in timed conditions. - Day 2: Review every miss; revisit relevant chapter sections. - Day 3: Re-take Chapter Review Questions for any chapter where you scored under 80%. - Day 4: Second full practice exam; aim for 80%+ overall. - Day 5: Review weakest 20% of items; targeted reading. - Day 6: Light review only; rest your brain. - Day 7 (exam day): Sleep well; arrive 30 minutes early.

.2 Eight-Week Distributed Plan (8–10 hours per week)

Weeks 1–2 — Chapter 1: Healthcare Industry, Roles, and Stakeholders - Read once carefully (3 hours). Build stakeholder map (1 hour). Complete review questions (1 hour). Repeat any missed rationales (1 hour). Practice five additional industry questions (2 hours).

Weeks 3–4 — Chapter 2: Technology Environment - Read once carefully (4 hours). Flashcards for HL7, FHIR, DICOM, X12 (2 hours). Build a separate flashcard set for ONC HTI-1 (DSI § 170.315(b)(11)), CMS Interoperability and Prior Authorization Final Rule, ASTP/ONC HTI-2, and TEFCA QHIN designation timeline (1 hour). Review questions and rationales (2 hours). Cumulative review of Chapters 1–2 (1 hour).

Week 5 — Chapter 3: Systems Analysis, Design, and Selection - Read (3 hours). SDLC phase/deliverable matrix from memory (1 hour). Review questions (2 hours). Two practice cases (vendor selection, workflow analysis) (2 hours).

Week 6 — Chapter 4: Implementation, Support, and Maintenance - Read (3 hours). ITIL practice flashcards (1 hour). Review questions (2 hours). Cutover strategy matrix from memory (1 hour). Joint Commission Sentinel Event Policy and HIT-related examples (0.5 hours). Mid-point practice (10 random questions) (0.5 hour).

Week 7 — Chapter 5: Privacy and Security - Read (4 hours). HIPAA rule and standards flashcards (1.5 hours). NIST publication crosswalk (0.5 hour). December 2024 HIPAA Security NPRM provisions, FIPS 140-2 EPCS citation, PCI DSS vs HIPAA scope, Section 1557 phased compliance dates (1 hour). Review questions (1 hour).

Week 8 — Chapter 6 and Final Drill - Read Chapter 6 (3 hours). EVM and change framework flashcards (1 hour). FDA PCCP for AI/ML SaMD (0.5 hour). Full 50-question practice exam (1.5 hours). Review every miss (2 hours). Light review and rest (final day).

Use any unused weekend hours each week for cumulative review; the most predictive practice is re-doing chapter review questions one week after first attempt and verifying the rationales remain clear.

Good luck. The CAHIMS credential is a credential of breadth — your goal is not to master any one domain, but to recognize the question type and the right framework within seconds. Build that recognition through repeated, deliberate practice with the rationales, and you will pass.

Full revised guide also saved to `/tmp/cahims_2026_revised.md` for convenience. All adversarial-reviewer corrections applied: reproductive health NPRM/Final Rule dates split (2023/2024), QHIN count corrected to 5 with CommonWell Feb 2024 added, DEA EPCS FIPS 140-2 citation per 21 CFR 1311.115, Practice Q21 and Q33 stems clarified, $4.9T attributed to 2023 NHE, "Regenstrein" corrected to "Regenstrief", speculative OCR-MFA statement replaced with factual December 2024 Security NPRM reference, HTI-1 phased compliance note added to US Core 3.1.1 paragraph, Section 1557 phased dates (May 1, 2025 for 45 CFR 92.210) added, HTI-1 DSI paragraph (§ 170.315(b)(11)) added, plus all seven missing topics integrated (HTI-1 DSI, Dec 2024 Security NPRM, CMS Interop/PA Final Rule, ASTP/ONC HTI-2, FDA PCCP, PCI DSS scope, Joint Commission Sentinel Event Policy).

Project Management and the Health IT Project Lifecycle

Exam Weight: Approximately 12–16 percent (integrated across Systems and Administration domains)

.3 Learning Objectives

After completing this chapter, the candidate will be able to:

- Describe the five PMBOK process groups and the triple constraint as they apply to health information technology projects.
- Explain the purpose and content of foundational project artifacts, including the project charter, scope statement, and work breakdown structure.
- Interpret common scheduling tools—Gantt charts, milestones, and the critical path—and construct a simple risk register and RACI matrix.
- Compare waterfall and Agile/Scrum delivery approaches and select the appropriate method for a given health IT initiative.
- Outline the phases of an electronic health record implementation, distinguish go-live models, and explain the role of post-implementation review.

.4 Why Project Management Matters in Health IT

Health information technology initiatives are rarely simple software installations. A typical **electronic health record (EHR)** implementation touches clinical workflows, billing systems, laboratory and pharmacy interfaces, medical devices, regulatory reporting, and the daily routines of physicians, nurses, registration clerks, and revenue-cycle staff. Because the stakes include patient safety, regulatory compliance, and tens of millions of dollars, disciplined **project management** is the discipline that keeps these efforts on scope, on schedule, and on budget while protecting quality.

Project management is defined by the Project Management Institute (PMI) as *the application of knowledge, skills, tools, and techniques to project activities to meet project requirements*. A **project** is a temporary endeavor undertaken to create a unique product, service, or result. The word *temporary* is important: every project has a defined beginning and end. This distinguishes a project (implementing a new patient portal) from **operations** (the ongoing daily support of that portal once it is live). The CAHIMS candidate should be able to recognize when an activity is project work and when it has transitioned into operational support and maintenance.

The person accountable for delivering the project is the **project manager (PM)**. In health IT settings, the PM coordinates among the IT department, clinical leadership, vendors, and end users. Larger programs are overseen by a **project management office (PMO)**, a centralized organizational unit that standardizes governance, templates, and reporting across many projects. A **program** is a group of related projects managed in a coordinated way—for example, an enterprise EHR modernization program might contain separate projects for the inpatient module, the ambulatory module, and the data-warehouse migration.

> **Key Concept**
>
> A project is *temporary and unique*; operations are *ongoing and repetitive*. Recognizing the transition point—often the moment of go-live and stabilization—helps the organization shift staff, budget, and accountability from the project team to the support team.

.5 The Five Process Groups and the Triple Constraint

PMI's *A Guide to the Project Management Body of Knowledge* (the **PMBOK Guide**) organizes project work into five **process groups**. These are not strictly sequential phases; they overlap and repeat, but they describe the logical flow of effort across a project's life.

1. **Initiating** — Authorizing the project and defining it at a high level. The major output is the **project charter**, which formally launches the project and names the project manager.
2. **Planning** — Establishing scope, refining objectives, and defining the course of action. This is typically the most document-intensive group, producing the scope statement, the work breakdown structure, the schedule, the budget, the communication plan, and the risk register.
3. **Executing** — Performing the work defined in the plan: configuring software, building interfaces, training users, and coordinating people and resources.
4. **Monitoring and Controlling** — Tracking progress against the plan, comparing actual performance to the baseline, and managing change. Status reports and change control happen here.
5. **Closing** — Formally finalizing the project, obtaining acceptance of deliverables, releasing resources, and documenting lessons learned.

These process groups interact with ten **knowledge areas** (integration, scope, schedule, cost, quality, resource, communications, risk, procurement, and stakeholder management). The CAHIMS candidate is not expected to memorize all forty-nine PMBOK processes, but should understand how the process groups map to the everyday rhythm of a health IT project.

Underlying every project is the **triple constraint**, sometimes called the **iron triangle** or **project management triangle**. The three competing constraints are:

- **Scope** — the work that must be done; the features and deliverables.
- **Time** — the schedule; how long the project will take.
- **Cost** — the budget; the resources required.

These three are interdependent. If a clinical sponsor adds new requirements (expanding **scope**) without extending the deadline or increasing funding, something must give—typically **quality** suffers or the team burns out. Modern practice places **quality** at the center of the triangle (or adds it as a fourth constraint), recognizing that changes to any side affect the quality of the result. A core PM skill is explaining these trade-offs to stakeholders: *We can add the new reporting module, but doing so will push go-live back three weeks or require two more analysts.*

> **Exam Tip**
>
> When a question describes a sponsor demanding more features with no additional time or money, the expected answer almost always involves managing the **triple constraint**—negotiating scope, schedule, or budget rather than silently absorbing the change. Unmanaged scope growth is called **scope creep.**

.6 Foundational Planning Artifacts: Charter, Scope Statement, and WBS

Three documents anchor the early life of any health IT project, and CAHIMS questions frequently test the ability to tell them apart.

The **project charter** is created during initiating. It is a short, authoritative document that *formally authorizes the project*, names and empowers the project manager, identifies the **sponsor** (the executive who funds and champions the project), states the high-level business need and objectives, and lists known constraints and assumptions. Without a charter, the PM has no formal authority to assign resources. The charter answers *why* the project exists and *who* is in charge.

The **scope statement** (part of the broader scope-management effort) comes during planning and is far more detailed. It defines the project and product **deliverables**, the **acceptance criteria** by which deliverables will be judged complete, and—critically—what is **out of scope**. Explicitly documenting exclusions ("the project will *not* include integration with the legacy radiology PACS") is one of the strongest defenses against scope creep. The scope statement answers *what* will be delivered.

The **work breakdown structure (WBS)** decomposes the total scope of work into smaller, manageable components. It is a hierarchical, deliverable-oriented breakdown: the top level is the project, the next levels are major deliverables or phases, and the lowest level contains **work packages**—chunks of work small enough to estimate, schedule, and assign. The smallest defined units of work are sometimes called **activities** or **tasks**. A guideline many PMs use is the **100 percent rule**: the WBS must capture 100 percent of the work defined in the scope, and no more. The WBS answers *how the work is organized*; it does not show timing or sequence, which is the job of the schedule.

A simple WBS fragment for an ambulatory EHR project might look like this:

```
1.0 Ambulatory EHR Implementation
    1.1 Project Management
    1.2 System Build and Configuration
        1.2.1 Provider templates
        1.2.2 Order sets
        1.2.3 Clinical decision support rules
    1.3 Interfaces
        1.3.1 Lab interface
        1.3.2 Pharmacy interface
    1.4 Testing
    1.5 Training
    1.6 Go-Live and Support
```

.7 Scheduling: Gantt Charts, Milestones, and the Critical Path

Once the WBS defines *what* work exists, the schedule sequences it in time. The most recognizable scheduling tool is the **Gantt chart**, a horizontal bar chart with tasks listed down the left side and a calendar across the top. Each task appears as a bar whose length represents its duration; bars are positioned to show start and finish dates, and connecting lines or arrows can show **dependencies** between tasks.

A **dependency** describes the relationship between two activities. The most common is **finish-to-start**: the lab interface cannot be tested until it has been built. Dependencies create chains of work. **Milestones** are zero-duration markers of significant events—"build complete," "user acceptance testing signed off," "go-live"—and are shown as diamonds on a Gantt chart. Milestones are useful for executive reporting because they communicate progress without overwhelming detail.

The **critical path** is the longest sequence of dependent activities through the project, and it determines the *shortest possible project duration*. Activities on the critical path have zero **float** (also called **slack**)—the amount of time an activity can slip without delaying the project. If a task on the critical path is late by one day, the entire project finishes one day later, unless time is recovered. Tasks *not* on the critical path have float and can absorb some delay without affecting the end date. The technique of identifying this path is the **critical path method (CPM)**.

For an entry-level associate, the key practical takeaways are: (1) watch critical-path tasks most closely because they offer no buffer; (2) a delay to a non-critical task does not necessarily delay the project; and (3) when the schedule must be compressed, the PM looks at the critical path first. Two compression techniques appear on exams: **fast tracking** (performing activities in parallel that were planned in sequence, which adds risk) and **crashing** (adding resources to critical-path tasks to shorten them, which adds cost).

> **Key Concept**
>
> The **critical path** is the longest path of dependent tasks and equals the shortest time in which the project can finish. Tasks on it have zero float, so a delay there delays the whole project.

.8 Stakeholders, the RACI Matrix, Resources, and Budget

A **stakeholder** is any individual or group that can affect, or is affected by, the project. In health IT, stakeholders include the executive sponsor, clinical leadership (the chief medical officer, chief nursing officer, and the **chief medical information officer (CMIO)**), physicians and nurses, registration and billing staff, IT analysts, the software vendor, compliance and privacy officers, and—indirectly—patients. **Stakeholder identification** happens early, often producing a **stakeholder register** that lists each party, their interest, their influence, and their communication needs. A common tool is the **power/interest grid**, which plots stakeholders by how much power and interest they have to determine how closely each should be managed.

Once stakeholders and tasks are known, the project must clarify *who does what.* The **RACI matrix** (also called a responsibility assignment matrix) maps people or roles against tasks using four designations:

- **R — Responsible:** the person(s) who perform the work.
- **A — Accountable:** the single person ultimately answerable for the task being completed correctly. There should be exactly one "A" per task.
- **C — Consulted:** people whose input is sought (two-way communication) before or during the work.
- **I — Informed:** people who are kept up to date on progress or outcomes (one-way communication).

A simplified RACI for an EHR training task might assign the training lead as Responsible, the project manager as Accountable, the clinical informatics nurse as Consulted, and unit managers as Informed. The CAHIMS candidate should remember the rule that **only one role is Accountable** for any given activity; diffuse accountability is a frequent source of project failure.

Resource management addresses the people, equipment, and materials the project needs. A **resource histogram** can show whether the team is over- or under-allocated across the schedule. **Budget basics** in PMBOK terms begin with estimating the cost of each work package and then aggregating those estimates into a **cost baseline**—the approved, time-phased budget against which spending is tracked. Costs include labor (often the largest line in a health IT project), software licenses, hardware, interface development, vendor professional services, and a **contingency reserve** set aside for identified risks. Tracking actual spend against the cost baseline is part of monitoring and controlling; a simple form of this is **earned value**, though associate-level candidates need only understand the concept that the project compares *planned cost, actual cost,* and *value of work completed* to judge financial health.

.9 Risk Management and the Risk Register

A **risk** is an uncertain event that, if it occurs, has a positive or negative effect on a project objective. In practice, health IT teams focus on **threats** (negative risks) such as interface failures, vendor delays, insufficient training, data-migration errors, and physician resistance, while remaining alert to **opportunities** (positive risks). Risk management is iterative: risks are identified, analyzed, planned for, and monitored throughout the project.

Risk identification uses techniques such as brainstorming, expert interviews, checklists from prior projects, and lessons-learned archives. Each identified risk is logged in a **risk register**, a living document that typically captures, for every risk: a description, the **probability** (likelihood of occurring), the **impact** (severity if it occurs), a combined **risk score** or priority, the **risk owner**, and the planned **response**.

The four classic **risk response strategies** for threats are:

- **Avoid** — eliminate the threat by changing the plan (for example, keeping a proven legacy interface rather than building a new, risky one).
- **Mitigate** — reduce the probability or impact (for example, adding extra testing cycles).
- **Transfer** — shift the impact to a third party (for example, contractual penalties on a vendor, or insurance).
- **Accept** — take no proactive action but, for active acceptance, hold a contingency reserve.

A simplified risk register row might read: *Risk: Pharmacy interface not ready by go-live. Probability: Medium. Impact: High. Score: High. Owner: Integration lead. Response: Mitigate—add parallel testing and a manual fallback workflow.* The CAHIMS candidate should be able to read such a register and identify the owner and response strategy.

> **Exam Tip**
>
> Memorize the four threat responses—**avoid, mitigate, transfer, accept**. A question that describes buying insurance or writing a vendor penalty clause is testing **transfer**. A question that describes adding extra testing is testing **mitigate**. A question that describes removing a risky feature entirely is testing **avoid.**

.10 Communication Planning and Status Reporting

Studies of project failure repeatedly cite poor communication as a root cause, and the PM spends a large share of time communicating. A **communication management plan** documents *who* needs *what* information, *when, in what format,* and *through what channel.* For a health IT project, the plan might specify a weekly written status report to the steering committee, a daily huddle for the build team, monthly executive dashboards, and an escalation path for urgent issues.

The number of potential communication channels grows rapidly with team size, following the formula $n(n - 1) / 2$, where n is the number of people. A team of five has ten channels; a team of ten has forty-five. This mathematical reality is one reason large projects formalize communication rather than relying on informal conversation.

A **status report** is the routine instrument of monitoring and controlling. Effective status reports are concise and compare actual progress to the baseline. A common format is **RAG status** (Red, Amber, Green), giving each major area a color: green means on track, amber means at risk and needs attention, and red means a problem requiring escalation. Status reports also surface the project's **issues** (problems that have already occurred and need resolution) as distinct from **risks** (problems that *might* occur). The distinction matters on exams: a risk that materializes becomes an issue. Issues are tracked in an **issue log** with an owner and a target resolution date.

Change control is the disciplined process for managing requests to alter scope, schedule, or budget. When a stakeholder requests a change, it is documented as a **change request**, evaluated for impact on the triple constraint, and approved or rejected by a **change control board (CCB)** before the project plan and baselines are updated. This formal process is what separates a managed scope adjustment from uncontrolled **scope creep.**

.11 Waterfall versus Agile/Scrum in Health IT

Health IT projects are delivered using one of two broad approaches, or a blend of both.

The **waterfall** (or **predictive**) approach proceeds through sequential phases—requirements, design, build, test, deploy—where each phase is largely completed before the next begins. Waterfall works best when requirements are stable and well understood, when heavy regulatory documentation is required, and when the deliverable is a defined, configurable system. A large EHR implementation with a fixed vendor product, firm go-live date, and extensive compliance documentation often follows a predominantly waterfall structure. Its weakness is inflexibility: discovering a requirement gap late in the project is expensive to fix.

The **Agile** approach, and its most common framework **Scrum**, delivers work in short, iterative cycles called **sprints** (typically one to four weeks). Rather than defining all requirements up front, Agile maintains a prioritized **product backlog**—a ranked list of features and requirements. The **product owner** owns and prioritizes the backlog; the **Scrum Master** facilitates the process and removes obstacles; the **development team** builds the product. Each sprint pulls items from the backlog into a **sprint backlog**, the team works to produce a potentially shippable increment, and the cycle includes a brief **sprint planning** session, a short daily **stand-up** (also called the **daily Scrum**, usually fifteen minutes, answering what was done, what is next, and what is blocking), a **sprint review** to demonstrate the increment, and a **sprint retrospective** to improve the process. Agile suits projects with evolving requirements, such as building a patient-facing mobile app, developing custom clinical decision support, or iterating on a data-analytics dashboard.

Many health systems adopt a **hybrid** model: the overall EHR program runs on a waterfall timeline with fixed milestones and go-live dates, while individual workstreams—report development, custom tools, optimization after go-live—use Agile sprints. The CAHIMS candidate should be able to match the approach to the situation: stable, regulated, fixed-scope work leans waterfall; evolving, exploratory, frequently changing work leans Agile.

> **Key Concept**
> In **Scrum**, the **product owner** prioritizes the backlog, the **Scrum Master** facilitates and clears obstacles, and the team self-organizes to deliver a working increment each **sprint**. The daily **stand-up** is a coordination meeting, not a status report to management.

.12 The EHR Implementation Project as a Worked Example

To see these concepts together, consider a community hospital implementing a new inpatient EHR. The project commonly moves through recognizable phases that map onto the process groups.

Planning and design follows charter approval. The team confirms scope, builds the WBS and schedule, identifies stakeholders, and—critically—conducts **workflow analysis** of current ("as-is") and future ("to-be") clinical processes. Decisions about how the system will be configured for the organization's specialties begin here.

Build and configuration is the executing-heavy phase where analysts construct provider templates, **order sets**, clinical decision support alerts, documentation flowsheets, and the data dictionary. This is followed by **interface development**, connecting the EHR to laboratory, radiology, pharmacy, and billing systems, often using **HL7** messaging standards.

Data migration and conversion moves selected historical patient data from legacy systems into the new EHR—an error-prone step that demands careful validation. **Testing** then proceeds in layers: **unit testing** of individual components, **integration testing** of connected systems and interfaces, and **user acceptance testing (UAT)** in which clinicians validate that the system supports real workflows. **End-to-end** testing traces a patient through registration, orders, results, documentation, and billing.

Training prepares end users, frequently using the **train-the-trainer** model in which a cadre of **super users**—clinical staff with deeper system knowledge—learn first and then teach and support their peers. Training is scheduled close to go-live so skills stay fresh.

The project then reaches **go-live**, after which it transitions into **stabilization** and ongoing operations. The discipline of carrying the same artifacts—WBS tasks, the risk register, the issue log, and the RACI—through every phase is what keeps a sprawling EHR project coherent.

.13 Go-Live Models and Support Structures

Selecting a **go-live model** is among the most consequential decisions in an EHR project, and CAHIMS questions test the contrast directly.

In a **big-bang** go-live, the entire organization (or a whole hospital) switches to the new system on a single cutover date, with the legacy system retired at once. The advantages are a single transition, no prolonged period of running two systems, and immediate organization-wide consistency. The disadvantages are concentrated risk—if something fails, it affects everyone at once—and the need for intense, all-hands support during the cutover.

In a **phased** (or **rolling**) go-live, the system is brought up incrementally—by location, by department, or by module—over weeks or months. This spreads risk and lets the team apply lessons from early waves to later ones, but it requires running old and new systems in parallel for a time (which can create reconciliation and interface complexity) and prolongs the overall transition. A related variant is the **pilot** go-live, in which one unit or clinic adopts the system first as a proof of concept before broader rollout.

Whatever the model, the period immediately after go-live demands heightened support. Two structures are standard. A **command center** is a centralized hub—physical or virtual—staffed by IT, clinical informatics, vendor representatives, and decision-makers who triage and resolve issues in real time, track them on a dashboard, and escalate quickly. **At-the-elbow support** places super users and trained support staff physically beside clinicians at the point of care during the first days of use, answering questions, correcting workflow missteps, and building user confidence. Together, the command center and at-the-elbow support form the safety net that carries an organization through the highest-risk window of the entire project.

> **Exam Tip**
>
> **Big-bang** = everyone at once (single cutover, concentrated risk). **Phased/rolling** = incremental rollout (spread risk, but parallel-system complexity). **Command center** = centralized issue triage; **at-the-elbow** = support physically next to end users at go-live.

.14 Closing the Project: Post-Implementation Review and Lessons Learned

A project is not finished when the system goes live; it is finished when it is formally **closed.** Closing includes obtaining final acceptance of deliverables from the sponsor, completing financial and contractual closeout with vendors, releasing the project team, and—most importantly for organizational learning—conducting a **post-implementation review (PIR).**

The PIR, sometimes called a **post-project review** or **post-mortem**, evaluates the project against its original objectives: Did it deliver the agreed scope? Was it on schedule and within budget? Did it achieve the intended

benefits realization—for example, reduced medication errors, faster documentation, or improved patient throughput? Benefits often cannot be measured until weeks or months after go-live, so the PIR may occur after a stabilization period.

The signature output of closing is the **lessons-learned** document. Lessons learned capture what went well, what went poorly, and what should be done differently next time, and they are archived in the organization's **knowledge base** (often maintained by the PMO) so future projects can draw on real experience rather than repeating mistakes. A lesson such as "data migration validation was under-resourced and caused a two-week delay" becomes a checklist item for the next implementation. The discipline of capturing and *reusing* lessons learned is what turns a series of individual projects into an organization that steadily gets better at delivering health IT.

For the CAHIMS candidate, the essential point is that closing is a deliberate, value-adding process group—not an afterthought. Skipping formal closure leaves deliverables unaccepted, vendors un-reconciled, and hard-won knowledge undocumented.

.15 Chapter 7 Review Questions

Q1. A clinical sponsor asks the project manager to add a new specialty documentation module to an EHR implementation that is already mid-build, but insists the go-live date and budget cannot change. According to project management principles, what is the project manager's most appropriate first action?

A) Quietly add the module and have the team work additional hours to absorb it
B) Refuse the request outright because the plan is already approved
C) Evaluate the change request's impact on the triple constraint and present the scope, schedule, and cost trade-offs
D) Immediately escalate the sponsor to the hospital board for discipline

Answer: C — Adding scope without adjusting time or cost stresses the **triple constraint**. The PM should process the request through change control, analyze its impact on scope, schedule, and cost (and quality), and present the trade-offs so an informed decision can be made. Silently absorbing it (A) invites scope creep and burnout; flatly refusing (B) or escalating punitively (D) are not sound change-management responses.

Q2. During schedule planning, a project manager identifies that the lab interface build, the lab interface testing, and the lab go-live tasks form the longest chain of dependent activities in the project, with no slack between them. What is this chain called, and what is its significance?

A) The work breakdown structure; it shows how work is organized
B) The critical path; a delay to any task on it delays the entire project
C) The communication plan; it shows who receives status reports
D) The risk register; it lists threats and their owners

Answer: B — The longest sequence of dependent tasks with zero float is the **critical path**, and it determines the shortest possible project duration. A delay to any critical-path task delays the whole project. The WBS (A) organizes work but shows no timing; the communication plan (C) and risk register (D) are unrelated artifacts.

Q3. On an EHR project's RACI matrix, the data-migration task lists the migration analyst as Responsible, the project manager as Accountable, the database vendor as Consulted, and several department managers as Informed. Which statement about this assignment is correct?

A) There should be multiple people marked Accountable to share responsibility
B) "Consulted" means the vendor only receives one-way updates after the work is done
C) Exactly one role should be Accountable, and "Informed" parties receive one-way communication about progress
D) The Responsible and Accountable designations always belong to the same person

Answer: C — In a RACI matrix, exactly one role should be **Accountable** for a given task, and **Informed** parties receive one-way updates. **Consulted** implies two-way input *before or during* the work, not after (ruling out B). Multiple Accountable parties (A) diffuse accountability, and Responsible and Accountable are frequently different people (ruling out D).

Q4. A hospital implementing a new EHR decides to bring the system live one department at a time over three months, applying lessons from each department to the next. Which go-live model does this describe, and what is a primary trade-off?

A) Big-bang; it concentrates all risk on a single cutover date

B) Phased/rolling; it spreads risk but requires running legacy and new systems in parallel for a time
C) Pilot; the entire organization adopts the system simultaneously
D) Command center; it places super users beside clinicians at the point of care

Answer: B — Bringing the system up incrementally by department is a **phased (rolling)** go-live, which spreads risk and allows learning between waves but requires running old and new systems in parallel, adding reconciliation and interface complexity. Big-bang (A) is a single simultaneous cutover; a pilot (C) is one unit first, not the whole organization at once; and a command center (D) is a support structure, not a go-live model.

Q5. Which of the following best describes the appropriate use of Agile/Scrum versus waterfall in a health IT setting?

A) Waterfall is always superior because health care is regulated, so Agile should never be used
B) Agile/Scrum, with sprints and a prioritized backlog, suits evolving requirements such as a custom analytics dashboard, while waterfall suits stable, well-defined, heavily documented work such as a fixed-scope EHR rollout
C) Agile eliminates the need for any planning, documentation, or stakeholder management
D) Scrum requires that all requirements be fully specified and frozen before any development begins

Answer: B — **Agile/Scrum** delivers in iterative **sprints** against a prioritized **backlog** and fits evolving, exploratory work; **waterfall** fits stable, well-understood, documentation-heavy efforts with fixed scope and dates. Many health systems blend the two. Agile is not always inferior (A), does not eliminate planning or stakeholder management (C), and—unlike waterfall—does *not* require freezing all requirements up front (D).

Clinical Informatics, Clinical Decision Support, and EHR Optimization

Exam Weight: Approximately 12–16 percent (Technology Environment and Clinical Systems)

.16 Learning Objectives

After completing this chapter, the candidate will be able to:

- Define clinical informatics and describe the role of the clinical informaticist as a bridge between clinicians and technical staff.
- Identify the core components of the electronic health record (EHR), including CPOE, eMAR, clinical documentation, results review, and the patient portal.
- Distinguish among the major types of clinical decision support (CDS) and apply the CDS "Five Rights" framework.
- Explain alert fatigue, its patient-safety consequences, and practical strategies to reduce it.
- Describe how data-quality anchors (problem list, medication reconciliation, allergy management) and standardized terminologies (SNOMED CT, LOINC, RxNorm, ICD-10-CM) support CDS and electronic clinical quality measures (eCQMs).

.17 What Clinical Informatics Is and Who Does It

Clinical informatics is the application of information technology and data science to the delivery of healthcare. It sits at the intersection of clinical practice, information systems, and the people and workflows that connect them. Where general health information technology focuses on the systems themselves, clinical informatics focuses on how those systems are used at the point of care to support safe, effective, and efficient patient care. A CAHIMS candidate should understand that informatics is not simply "running the EHR" — it is the disciplined study and improvement of how clinical information flows into, through, and out of the technology environment.

The practitioner who specializes in this work is the **clinical informaticist** (sometimes called a clinical informatics specialist or clinical analyst). This individual serves as a **bridge** or translator between two communities that often speak different languages: the clinicians who care for patients and the technical teams who build and maintain the systems. A nurse, pharmacist, physician, or other clinician who moves into an informatics role brings domain knowledge of how care actually happens, then learns enough about system configuration, data structures, and project methods to specify what the technology must do. Physician leaders in this space frequently hold the title **Chief Medical Information Officer (CMIO)**, and nursing leaders the title **Chief Nursing Information Officer (CNIO)**. These executive roles partner with the **Chief Information Officer (CIO)** to set strategy, but the day-to-day translation work is done by analysts and specialists embedded with clinical departments.

The value of the informaticist is most visible during system **selection, build, optimization, and governance.** When a hospital chooses a new EHR or adds a module, the informaticist gathers clinical requirements, validates that proposed workflows match real practice, and tests the build before it reaches patients. After go-live, the informaticist responds to enhancement requests, investigates safety events involving the system, and proposes optimization. Because this person understands both worlds, they can prevent a common failure mode: a technically correct build that no clinician can actually use, or a clinician request that, if built literally, would create a safety hazard.

> **Key Concept**
>
> Clinical informatics is fundamentally a translation discipline. The clinical informaticist converts clinical intent into system requirements and converts system constraints back into language clinicians can act on. Hiring clinicians into these roles is deliberate — domain credibility is what makes the translation trustworthy.

.18 Core Components of the EHR

The modern **electronic health record (EHR)** is a suite of integrated functions rather than a single screen. For the CAHIMS exam, candidates should be able to name the core components and state the purpose of each.

Computerized Provider Order Entry (CPOE) is the function through which authorized clinicians enter orders — for medications, laboratory tests, imaging, diets, referrals, and other care — directly into the system. CPOE replaced handwritten and verbal orders, and its primary patient-safety contribution is the elimination of transcription errors and illegible handwriting. CPOE is also the entry point where many decision-support checks fire, because the order is captured in structured, computable form at the moment it is created.

The **electronic Medication Administration Record (eMAR)** is the nursing-facing complement to CPOE. After a medication is ordered, verified by pharmacy, and dispensed, the eMAR documents the administration: who gave the drug, what dose, by what route, and at what time. When paired with **barcode medication administration (BCMA)**, the nurse scans the patient's wristband and the medication barcode to confirm the **"five rights" of medication administration** (right patient, right drug, right dose, right route, right time) before the dose is given. The eMAR plus BCMA closes the loop from order to administration and is one of the strongest safety controls in inpatient care.

Clinical documentation captures the narrative and structured record of care — progress notes, history and physical, nursing assessments, flowsheets, and discharge summaries. Documentation increasingly uses **templates** and structured data entry so that information can be reused for orders, decision support, billing, and quality measurement rather than locked inside free text.

Results review is the component clinicians use to retrieve and interpret laboratory values, imaging reports, pathology, and other diagnostic results. Good results-review design surfaces abnormal and critical values clearly, supports trending over time, and routes results to the responsible provider for acknowledgment.

The **patient portal** extends the EHR to patients and caregivers. It typically offers secure messaging, appointment scheduling, access to test results, visit summaries, medication lists, and bill payment. Under the federal **information-blocking** requirements of the 21st Century Cures Act, patients now expect timely electronic access to most of their data, and the portal is the primary delivery channel. The CAHIMS candidate should understand the portal both as a patient-engagement tool and as a compliance touchpoint.

These components share a single **integrated database**, which is what distinguishes an EHR from a collection of standalone systems. Because an order placed in CPOE, the resulting administration in the eMAR, the supporting note in documentation, and the confirming lab in results review all reference the same patient record, the system can reason across them — and that shared data is the foundation for decision support.

.19 Clinical Decision Support: Types and Purposes

Clinical decision support (CDS) is functionality that provides clinicians, staff, and patients with knowledge and person-specific information, intelligently filtered and presented at appropriate times, to improve care. CDS is not a single feature; it is a family of intervention types, and the exam expects candidates to distinguish them.

Alerts (also called interruptive alerts or pop-ups) interrupt the workflow to warn of a potential problem — a drug-drug interaction, a drug-allergy conflict, a duplicate order, a dose outside safe limits, or an abnormal value. Alerts are powerful but costly to clinician attention, which is why their design and tuning matter so much (see Section 8.4).

Order sets group related orders into a single, evidence-based bundle that a clinician can review and place together — for example, an admission order set for community-acquired pneumonia that includes appropriate antibiotics, labs, and monitoring. Order sets embed best practice into the workflow without interrupting it, and they speed ordering while improving consistency.

Care plans (and clinical pathways) lay out a coordinated, multidisciplinary sequence of interventions over an episode of care, helping teams follow evidence-based protocols and track progress toward goals.

Documentation templates structure note-writing so that required elements are captured and so that discrete data is recorded for reuse. A well-built template prompts the clinician for the right information without forcing irrelevant fields.

Reminders prompt clinicians or patients about care that is due but not yet done — an overdue immunization, a needed diabetic foot exam, a cancer screening. Reminders typically appear as non-interruptive indicators (a health-maintenance banner, a care-gap list) rather than blocking pop-ups.

Infobuttons are context-sensitive links that retrieve reference knowledge relevant to whatever the clinician is viewing — for example, a small icon next to a medication that opens a monograph, or next to a diagnosis that opens evidence summaries. Infobuttons follow the **HL7 Infobutton standard**, which lets the EHR pass context (drug, problem, lab) to an external knowledge resource.

Beyond these, CDS includes **smart documentation**, **relevant-data presentation** (dashboards and summaries that organize information for a decision), and **calculators** (risk scores such as a sepsis score or a bleeding-risk score). The common thread is that CDS turns raw data plus medical knowledge into actionable guidance at the point of decision.

> **Exam Tip**
>
> When a question describes a CDS scenario, identify the *type* before judging it. Interruptive alerts and non-interruptive reminders solve different problems. An exam item that asks how to reduce interruptions without losing safety value is usually pointing toward converting a low-value alert into a passive reminder or an order-set default rather than removing the logic entirely.

.20 The CDS Five Rights and Alert Fatigue

The most important design framework in CDS is the **"Five Rights"** of clinical decision support. To improve care, a CDS intervention must deliver:

1. **The right information** — evidence-based, specific to the situation, and actionable rather than generic.
2. **To the right person** — the team member who can act on it (a pharmacist, a nurse, the ordering physician, or the patient), not just whoever happens to be at the screen.
3. **In the right format** — the right intervention type, such as an order-set default, a reminder, an infobutton, or an interruptive alert, matched to how disruptive the situation warrants.
4. **Through the right channel** — the right delivery mechanism, such as the EHR, a patient-portal message, a mobile alert, or a printed handout.
5. **At the right time in the workflow** — the moment in the process where the information can change a decision, most often during ordering or documentation rather than after the fact.

A CDS intervention that fails any one of the Five Rights tends to fail overall. Correct information delivered to the wrong person, at the wrong moment, or in an overly disruptive format will be ignored, overridden, or worked around. The Five Rights give an organization a structured way to critique and redesign interventions.

The clearest failure mode of poorly designed alerts is **alert fatigue** — the desensitization that occurs when clinicians face so many alerts, many of them low-value or irrelevant, that they begin to dismiss them reflexively. Override rates for interruptive medication alerts frequently exceed 90 percent in published studies, which means the great majority of interruptions add cost without changing behavior. The danger is not merely annoyance: when clinicians click through alerts automatically, they may dismiss the rare alert that truly mattered, producing a patient-safety event. Alert fatigue is therefore both a usability problem and a safety problem.

Strategies to reduce alert fatigue are a favorite exam topic. Effective approaches include: **tiering alerts by severity** so that only high-risk situations interrupt while lower-risk information is presented passively; **suppressing duplicate and nuisance alerts** (for example, not re-firing an interaction the clinician already overrode in the same encounter); **increasing specificity** so alerts account for patient context such as renal function, age, or existing tolerance; **routing alerts to the right role** so a pharmacy-actionable alert goes to pharmacy rather than the prescriber; **requiring a reason for override** on the highest-severity alerts to preserve their weight; and **monitoring override and firing data** so the CDS governance team can retire or retune low-value rules. The goal is fewer, smarter interruptions — not the removal of safety logic.

> **Key Concept**
>
> More alerts do not equal more safety. Past a threshold, additional interruptive alerts reduce safety by training clinicians to dismiss them. The mature organization measures alert burden and override rates and continuously tunes its rules, treating alert design as an ongoing governance activity rather than a one-time build.

.21 Data-Quality Anchors and Standardized Terminologies

CDS is only as good as the data it reasons over. Three structured elements act as **data-quality anchors** because so many decision-support rules depend on them being accurate and current.

The **problem list** is the maintained, structured record of a patient's active diagnoses and significant conditions. A current problem list drives reminders (a diabetic patient triggers diabetic care-gap logic), order sets, and quality measures. A stale or duplicated problem list — full of resolved conditions or inconsistent entries — degrades every downstream rule. Maintaining the problem list is a shared clinical responsibility, and informatics teams design workflows that prompt clinicians to reconcile it.

Medication reconciliation is the process of comparing the medications a patient is actually taking against the medications ordered at each transition of care — admission, transfer, and discharge — to prevent omissions, duplications, dosing errors, and dangerous interactions. Because transitions are where medication errors cluster, reconciliation is both a Joint Commission **National Patient Safety Goal** and the data source that keeps the active medication list trustworthy for interaction checking.

Allergy management captures patient allergies and intolerances in a coded, structured form so that drug-allergy checking can fire correctly. An allergy recorded only as free text (for example, "sulfa — rash" typed into a note) cannot drive an automated alert; it must be coded to a recognized allergen concept. Distinguishing true allergies from intolerances and side effects also matters, because over-coding intolerances as allergies generates false alerts and contributes to alert fatigue.

For any of these anchors to feed automated logic, the data must be expressed in **standardized clinical terminologies** rather than local free text. The CAHIMS candidate should recognize the major vocabularies at an introductory level:

- **SNOMED CT** (Systematized Nomenclature of Medicine — Clinical Terms) is the comprehensive clinical terminology used for problems, diagnoses, findings, and procedures. It is the preferred vocabulary for the **problem list** and supports CDS reasoning across clinical concepts.
- **LOINC** (Logical Observation Identifiers Names and Codes) standardizes the names of **laboratory tests and clinical observations** — what was measured. LOINC lets results from different labs map to a common identifier so that trending and decision support work across sources.
- **RxNorm** provides normalized names and identifiers for **medications**, linking the many brand and generic names of a drug to a common concept. RxNorm underpins drug-interaction and drug-allergy checking and supports interoperable medication lists.
- **ICD-10-CM** (International Classification of Diseases, Tenth Revision, Clinical Modification) is the code set used primarily for **billing, reimbursement, and statistical reporting** of diagnoses. While SNOMED CT is preferred for clinical documentation and reasoning, ICD-10-CM is what claims and many quality reports require, and the EHR often maps between the two.

A useful way to remember the division of labor: **SNOMED CT for problems and findings, LOINC for what was measured (labs/observations), RxNorm for medications, and ICD-10-CM for billing diagnoses.** These vocabularies are the machine-readable substrate that makes alerts, reminders, and quality measures possible. They are also central to **interoperability**: standards such as HL7 FHIR and the United States Core Data for Interoperability (USCDI) reference these terminologies so that data exchanged between organizations remains computable.

> **Exam Tip**
>
> Match the terminology to its domain. If a question asks which standard codes laboratory results, the answer is LOINC, not ICD-10-CM. If it asks which is preferred for the clinical problem list, the answer is SNOMED CT. ICD-10-CM is the "billing/claims diagnosis" answer; RxNorm is the "medication" answer. Distinguishing these four is among the most reliably tested factual clusters in this domain.

.22 Clinical Quality Measures and How EHR Data Feeds Them

Electronic clinical quality measures (eCQMs) are standardized measures of healthcare quality that are calculated automatically from data already captured in the EHR — for example, the percentage of patients with diabetes whose blood pressure is controlled, or the percentage of eligible patients who received a recommended screening. eCQMs are central to value-based programs and to federal reporting under the **Medicare Promoting Interoperability** programs (the successor to the earlier Meaningful Use initiative) and the **Merit-based Incentive Payment System (MIPS).**

The critical insight for the CAHIMS candidate is that eCQMs depend entirely on **structured, coded EHR data.** An eCQM that measures controlled blood pressure can only count a patient if the blood-pressure reading was captured as discrete data, if the diabetes diagnosis is on the coded problem list, and if any exclusions (such as documented contraindications) are recorded in computable form. If clinicians document those facts only in free-text narrative, the measure cannot "see" them, and the organization's performance will appear worse than the care actually delivered. This is why informatics teams invest so heavily in templates, structured order entry, and terminology mapping — accurate measurement is a byproduct of capturing the right data in the right fields.

eCQMs are defined using standardized specifications — the **Clinical Quality Language (CQL)** expresses the logic, and **value sets** (curated lists of codes drawn from SNOMED CT, LOINC, RxNorm, ICD-10-CM, and other vocabularies) define which coded entries qualify. When an EHR is certified for quality reporting, it is tested against these specifications so that the same measure yields comparable results across organizations. The informaticist's role is to ensure the local build maps documentation and orders to the value sets the measures expect, then to validate that reported numbers reflect reality before submission.

The link back to decision support is direct: the same coded data that feeds an eCQM can also drive a **reminder** to close the gap before the visit ends. A care-gap reminder that a screening is overdue and the eCQM that later reports whether the screening was done are two views of the same underlying data. Well-designed organizations align their CDS and their quality measures so that the system both prompts the right care and accurately measures it.

.23 Usability, EHR Optimization, and Clinical Content Governance

After an EHR is live, the work shifts from implementation to continuous improvement. **Usability** — how effectively, efficiently, and satisfyingly clinicians can accomplish their tasks in the system — has emerged as a major determinant of safety, quality, and clinician well-being. Poor usability contributes to **clinician burnout**, documentation burden, and workarounds that bypass safety controls. Recognizing this, organizations now treat usability as a measurable property and conduct **EHR optimization** programs to improve it.

EHR optimization is the structured review and refinement of an already-deployed system. Typical activities include **workflow review** (observing how clinicians actually use the system and finding friction), simplifying overly long documentation templates, retuning alerts, redesigning order sets to match current evidence, building personalization tools such as user-specific order preferences, and retiring build that is no longer used. Optimization is data-informed: teams analyze system usage logs, alert override rates, note length, and time-in-system metrics to target the highest-impact changes. The defining feature is that optimization is **ongoing** — the EHR is never "done," because medicine, regulation, and workflows keep changing.

Because many people across an organization want changes to the EHR, those requests must be controlled through **clinical content governance.** Governance is the formal structure of committees, roles, and processes that decides which build requests are approved, how they are prioritized, who has authority to change shared clinical content (order sets, alerts, templates, CDS rules), and how changes are tested and released. A typical governance model includes a **CDS or clinical content committee** with clinical, pharmacy, informatics, and IT representation; defined **intake and prioritization** of enhancement requests; **standardized build and testing** before changes reach production; and **ongoing monitoring** of the content's effect. Governance prevents two opposite failures: uncontrolled local changes that fragment a shared system and create safety risk, and paralysis in which no improvement ever ships. For shared, safety-critical content like alerts and order sets, governance also ensures that a change requested by one department does not inadvertently harm another.

A specific governance responsibility is the **management of build requests.** Not every clinician request should be built as asked. The informaticist and governance body evaluate each request for safety, evidence, downstream effects, maintenance burden, and alignment with standards. A request to add yet another interruptive alert, for instance, may be better served by an order-set change or a passive reminder — and it is governance that makes that determination consistently rather than case by case at an individual analyst's discretion.

.24 Downtime Procedures and Data Integrity

Because clinical care cannot stop when the EHR is unavailable, every organization must maintain **downtime procedures** — the agreed plans and tools for continuing safe care during planned or unplanned system outages. Downtime may be **planned** (scheduled maintenance, upgrades) or **unplanned** (hardware failure, network outage, power loss, or a cyber event such as ransomware). The CAHIMS candidate should understand both the operational and the data-integrity dimensions.

Operationally, organizations rely on **business continuity** tools. A common control is a **read-only "downtime computer" or business-continuity server** that holds a recent snapshot of patient data so clinicians can still see medications, allergies, problems, and recent results when the live system is down. Paper **downtime forms** (paper MAR, paper order sheets, paper documentation) provide a way to continue documenting and ordering. Staff must be trained in advance and the forms kept current, because a downtime is the worst time to discover that procedures are stale.

The harder challenge is **data integrity** during and after the outage. Care delivered on paper during downtime must be **back-entered** (reconciled) into the EHR once it returns, accurately and with correct timestamps, so the record is complete and so that decision support and quality measures operate on real data. Recovery procedures must guard against lost orders, duplicate entries, and medications given on paper but never reconciled into the eMAR. Strong organizations define explicit **recovery and reconciliation** steps, assign responsibility for back-entry, and audit completeness afterward.

Downtime planning intersects directly with **privacy, security, and disaster recovery** (Chapter 5). The rise of ransomware has made extended unplanned downtime a realistic scenario, sometimes lasting days or weeks, which raises the stakes for robust paper procedures, current backups, and well-rehearsed recovery. For the exam, remember that downtime procedures are a **patient-safety and data-integrity control**, not merely an IT inconvenience — their purpose is to keep care safe when the technology is unavailable and to ensure the record is accurate once it returns.

> **Key Concept**
> The EHR will be unavailable at some point — the only question is whether the organization is prepared. Mature downtime planning has three parts: continue care safely (read-only access plus paper tools), preserve the data created during the outage, and reconcile that data accurately into the record afterward so that integrity, decision support, and quality measurement are not compromised.

.25 Chapter 8 Review Questions

Q1. A hospital is redesigning a drug-drug interaction alert that clinicians override more than 95 percent of the time. The clinical content committee wants to preserve safety value while reducing interruptions. Which approach is MOST consistent with the CDS "Five Rights" and alert-fatigue best practice?

A) Remove all drug-drug interaction logic from the system to eliminate the interruptions entirely.
B) Tier the alerts by severity so only high-risk interactions interrupt, route pharmacy-actionable alerts to pharmacy, and present lower-risk information passively.
C) Add a second confirmation pop-up after each override to slow clinicians down.
D) Convert every interaction alert into a hard stop that cannot be overridden.

Answer: B — Tiering by severity, routing alerts to the right person, and using passive presentation for lower-risk information directly applies the Five Rights (right person, right format, right time) and is the recommended way to cut alert burden without discarding safety logic. Removing all logic (A) eliminates safety value; adding friction (C) worsens fatigue; universal hard stops (D) are unsafe and impractical for low-risk interactions.

Q2. A clinical informaticist is mapping data so that automated decision support and quality measures function correctly. Which terminology is the preferred standard for coding entries on the patient's clinical problem list?

A) ICD-10-CM
B) LOINC
C) SNOMED CT
D) RxNorm

Answer: C — SNOMED CT is the preferred terminology for clinical problems, diagnoses, and findings and supports CDS reasoning. ICD-10-CM (A) is used primarily for billing and statistical reporting; LOINC (B) codes laboratory and observation results; RxNorm (D) codes medications.

Q3. During an unplanned EHR outage, nurses document medication administration on paper. After the system is restored, which action is MOST important to protect data integrity and downstream safety logic?

A) Discard the paper records once the system is back online to avoid duplication.
B) Wait until the next scheduled maintenance window to enter the paper data.

C) Accurately back-enter and reconcile the downtime documentation into the EHR with correct information and timestamps.
D) Leave the downtime period blank in the EHR because the paper record is the legal record.

Answer: C — Care delivered on paper must be accurately back-entered and reconciled into the EHR so the record is complete and so decision support and quality measures operate on real data. Discarding records (A) and leaving gaps (D) destroy integrity; delaying entry (B) leaves the record dangerously incomplete in the interim.

Q4. A quality team reports that the organization's eCQM for controlled blood pressure shows poor performance, even though clinicians believe their care is excellent. An informaticist reviews charts and finds that many blood-pressure readings are recorded only in free-text progress notes. What is the BEST explanation?
A) The eCQM specification is incorrect and should be ignored.
B) eCQMs are calculated from structured, coded data, so readings captured only as free text are not counted by the measure.
C) Blood pressure is not a valid quality measure in any federal program.
D) The patient portal is preventing the data from being counted.

Answer: B — eCQMs depend on structured, coded EHR data. Readings buried in free text cannot be computed by the measure, so performance appears worse than the care actually delivered. The fix is to capture the data discretely. The specification is standardized (A), blood-pressure control is a recognized measure (C), and the portal is unrelated to measure calculation (D).

Q5. A clinician requests that a new interruptive alert be added to warn about a specific situation. According to clinical content governance principles, what should happen to this request?
A) Any analyst should build it immediately, since the requesting clinician knows the clinical need best.
B) The request should be evaluated by the governance process for safety, evidence, downstream effects, and whether a less disruptive intervention (such as an order-set change or passive reminder) would better serve the need.
C) The request should be automatically denied because no new alerts are ever permitted.
D) The request should be forwarded directly to the EHR vendor to build.

Answer: B — Clinical content governance exists to evaluate build requests for safety, evidence, downstream impact, and maintenance burden, and to determine whether a less disruptive intervention is more appropriate for shared, safety-critical content. Immediate unilateral build (A) fragments a shared system and risks safety; blanket denial (C) prevents legitimate improvement; routing straight to the vendor (D) bypasses internal governance and local validation.

Healthcare Data Analytics, Reporting, and Dashboards

Exam Weight: Approximately 10–14 percent (Data and Analytics)

.26 Learning Objectives

After completing this chapter, the candidate will be able to:

- Explain the data–information–knowledge–wisdom (DIKW) hierarchy and distinguish among descriptive, diagnostic, predictive, and prescriptive analytics.
- Identify the major sources of healthcare data and differentiate structured from unstructured data.
- Describe foundational database concepts—relational tables, primary and foreign keys, and the purpose of SQL—along with data warehouses, data marts, and ETL.
- Differentiate operational reports from analytic dashboards, select appropriate key performance indicators, and apply data visualization best practices.
- Define the core dimensions of data quality and explain the role of data governance, data stewardship, and a data dictionary.

.27 From Data to Wisdom: The DIKW Hierarchy

Healthcare generates staggering volumes of data, but raw data alone changes nothing. The **DIKW hierarchy**—data, information, knowledge, wisdom—is the conceptual ladder that informatics professionals use to describe how raw measurements become actionable insight. Understanding this progression is foundational because nearly every analytics activity is, at root, an attempt to move a healthcare organization up the ladder.

At the base sits **data**: discrete, raw, unprocessed facts with no inherent meaning. A blood pressure reading of "148/92," a charge code, or a timestamp are all data points. They are accurate but isolated. The next rung is **information**, which is data placed in context and organized so it answers a question. "Patient Jones's blood pressure was 148/92 at 09:14 on Tuesday, up from 122/78 last week" is information—the same numbers, but now structured, related, and meaningful.

The third level is **knowledge**, which synthesizes information with experience, rules, and patterns to support understanding. Recognizing that "a rising blood pressure trend in a patient on this medication regimen suggests non-adherence or dosing problems" is knowledge. It draws on clinical evidence and accumulated experience. At the apex is **wisdom**, the appropriate and ethical application of knowledge to make sound decisions—knowing not just what the data say but what to *do*, and whether to act at all. Wisdom is the judgment to intervene, to wait, or to escalate.

For the CAHIMS candidate, the practical lesson is that analytics infrastructure exists to accelerate the climb from data to wisdom. Dashboards, reports, and registries are not ends in themselves; they are tools that compress the distance between a recorded fact and a defensible decision.

> **Key Concept**
>
> The DIKW hierarchy ascends from raw, context-free *data* to *information* (data in context), to *knowledge* (information plus experience and pattern), to *wisdom* (the ethical, appropriate application of knowledge to act). Each level adds context and judgment, not merely volume.

.28 The Four Types of Analytics

Healthcare analytics is conventionally divided into four maturity levels, each answering a different question and demanding more sophistication than the last. Candidates should be able to match an analytic activity to its type.

Descriptive analytics answers "What happened?" It summarizes historical data into reports, counts, averages, and rates. Monthly admission counts, average length of stay, and a quarterly tally of patient falls are all descriptive. This is the most common and accessible form of analytics, and the backbone of operational reporting. Most of the reports a hospital runs every day are descriptive.

Diagnostic analytics answers "Why did it happen?" It drills into data to find causes and relationships—using techniques such as root-cause analysis, drill-down, and correlation. If readmissions spiked in March, diagnostic analytics examines which units, diagnoses, or discharge processes were associated with the increase. It moves from observation toward explanation.

Predictive analytics answers "What is likely to happen?" It uses statistical models and machine learning trained on historical data to forecast future events. A sepsis-risk score, a 30-day readmission probability, or a no-show prediction for an appointment slot are predictive outputs. Predictive models produce probabilities, not certainties, and their value depends heavily on the quality of the training data and ongoing validation.

Prescriptive analytics answers "What should we do about it?" It is the most advanced level, recommending specific actions and often weighing trade-offs among options. A staffing-optimization tool that recommends nurse allocations given predicted census, or a clinical decision support rule that suggests a specific intervention, edges into prescriptive territory. Prescriptive analytics frequently builds on predictive outputs and incorporates constraints and goals.

A useful exam frame: the four types form a continuum of increasing complexity and increasing business value—descriptive (hindsight), diagnostic (insight), predictive (foresight), and prescriptive (decision support). Most healthcare organizations are strongest in descriptive and diagnostic analytics and are still maturing in the predictive and prescriptive tiers.

> **Exam Tip**
>
> Memorize the four questions: descriptive = "What happened?", diagnostic = "Why did it happen?", predictive = "What will happen?", prescriptive = "What should we do?" The exam often presents a scenario and asks you to classify the analytic type.

.29 Sources and Forms of Healthcare Data

Effective analytics depends on knowing where data originate and in what form they arrive. Healthcare data come from a wide and growing set of sources, and the CAHIMS candidate should recognize each.

The **electronic health record (EHR)** is the richest single source, holding clinical documentation, orders, results, medications, vital signs, and problem lists. **Administrative and claims data**—generated for billing and reimbursement—capture diagnoses (coded in ICD-10-CM), procedures (CPT and ICD-10-PCS), and charges; claims data are broad in population coverage but limited in clinical depth and subject to coding for payment rather than precision. **Registries**, such as cancer registries or device and immunization registries, aggregate standardized data on specific conditions or populations for surveillance, quality reporting, and research. **Health information exchanges (HIE)** supply data shared across organizations, giving a more complete longitudinal view of a patient who receives care in multiple settings. **Patient-generated health data (PGHD)**—from wearables, home monitoring devices, patient portals, and questionnaires—is a fast-growing source that originates with the patient rather than the provider. Additional sources include laboratory and imaging systems, pharmacy systems, public health feeds, and increasingly social determinants of health data drawn from community and survey sources.

Data also arrive in two broad forms. **Structured data** is organized into defined fields with predictable formats—a lab value, a coded diagnosis, a date of birth, a checkbox. Because each element lives in a known place with a known type, structured data is readily counted, filtered, and aggregated, making it the easiest to analyze. **Unstructured data** has no predefined model: free-text clinical notes, dictated reports, emails, scanned documents, and images. Estimates commonly cited in the informatics literature hold that the large majority—frequently put at roughly 80 percent—of healthcare data is unstructured. Unstructured data is rich but difficult to analyze directly; extracting meaning from it requires techniques such as **natural language processing (NLP)** to identify and code concepts buried in narrative text. **Semi-structured data**, such as an HL7 or FHIR message that carries tags but allows free text within fields, sits between the two.

The practical implication is that analytics teams spend enormous effort transforming heterogeneous, partly unstructured source data into clean, structured, analyzable form—work that precedes any chart or model.

.30 Database Foundations: Tables, Keys, and SQL

Behind every report and dashboard sits a database. CAHIMS does not require database administration skills, but it does expect conceptual fluency in how healthcare data is stored and retrieved.

Most operational healthcare systems use **relational databases**, which organize data into **tables** (also called relations). A table is a grid of **rows** (records) and **columns** (fields or attributes). A "Patients" table might have one row per patient and columns for patient ID, name, date of birth, and sex. An "Encounters" table might have one row per visit. Relational design deliberately splits data across multiple related tables rather than piling everything into one giant table—a principle related to **normalization**, which reduces redundancy and prevents inconsistencies.

Tables are linked through **keys**. A **primary key** is a column (or combination of columns) whose value uniquely identifies each row in a table—no two rows share the same value, and it is never empty. A patient's medical record number can serve as the primary key of the Patients table. A **foreign key** is a column in one table that refers to the primary key of another table, establishing a relationship between them. The Encounters table would carry a patient ID as a foreign key, linking each visit back to exactly one patient. These key relationships are what allow data scattered across many tables to be recombined coherently.

To retrieve and combine that data, analysts use **SQL (Structured Query Language)**, the standard language for relational databases. At a conceptual level—candidates need recognition, not coding mastery—three ideas matter. A **SELECT** statement chooses which columns to return ("SELECT patient_name, admit_date"). A **WHERE** clause filters which rows qualify ("WHERE admit_date is in the last 30 days"), so the query returns only the records that meet a condition. A **JOIN** combines rows from two or more tables based on a related key—joining Patients to Encounters on patient ID, for example, so a single result set can show patient names alongside their visits. The exam may ask you to recognize that a JOIN is the mechanism for connecting related tables, that a primary key uniquely identifies rows, and that a foreign key creates the link between tables. Mastery of SQL syntax is not expected; conceptual recognition is.

.31 Warehouses, Marts, and ETL

Operational databases—the live systems that run the EHR, lab, and billing—are optimized for fast transactions: admitting a patient, posting a result, recording a charge. They are not well suited to large analytic queries, which would slow the live system and which need data combined from many sources over long periods. The solution is a separate analytic environment.

A **data warehouse** is a large, central repository that integrates data from many operational source systems into a structure optimized for reporting and analysis. It is typically organized to hold historical, subject-oriented data—pulling clinical, financial, and administrative data into one consistent place so that analysts can ask cross-cutting questions without touching production systems. The **enterprise data warehouse (EDW)** is the organization-wide version of this concept and is a central piece of infrastructure in mature healthcare analytics programs.

A **data mart** is a smaller, focused subset of a warehouse, scoped to a single department, subject area, or use case—a quality data mart, a financial data mart, or an oncology data mart. Data marts make access faster and simpler for a particular audience and can be built either as carved-out pieces of a larger warehouse or as standalone stores.

Data does not move into a warehouse by itself; it gets there through **ETL—Extract, Transform, Load**. In the **extract** step, data is pulled from each source system. In the **transform** step—the most labor-intensive—it is cleaned, standardized, deduplicated, mapped to common code sets, and reshaped so that, for example, "M/F," "Male/Female," and "1/2" all become a single consistent representation. In the **load** step, the transformed data is written into the warehouse. A related modern variant, **ELT (Extract, Load, Transform)**, loads raw data first and transforms it inside the target platform; candidates should recognize the acronym but ETL is the classic model. The quality and discipline of the ETL process directly determine the trustworthiness of every downstream report, which is why ETL and data quality are tightly linked.

.32 Reports, Dashboards, and Choosing the Right KPIs

Once data is integrated, it must be delivered to people who will act on it—and the form of delivery matters. The exam distinguishes between two delivery modes.

An **operational report** is typically detailed, often row-level, scheduled or run on demand, and designed to support day-to-day work. A daily census list, a missing-charge report, an open-orders worklist, or a roster of patients due for follow-up are operational reports. They are frequently static, printed or exported, and answer concrete tactical questions for frontline staff.

An **analytic dashboard**, by contrast, presents summarized, visual, often interactive information—charts, gauges, and trend lines—designed to give a quick, at-a-glance view of performance and to support monitoring and decision-making. Dashboards typically aggregate data into indicators rather than listing individual records, refresh on a defined cadence, and let users drill down from a summary into detail. A useful distinction: operational reports tend to be detailed and transactional ("here are the rows"), while dashboards are summarized and indicator-driven ("here is how we are doing"). A related artifact, the **scorecard**, compares performance against predefined targets or benchmarks and is often associated with strategic frameworks such as the balanced scorecard.

Both reports and dashboards are organized around **key performance indicators (KPIs)**—the specific, measurable metrics an organization tracks to gauge progress toward its goals. Not every number is a KPI; a KPI is chosen deliberately because it reflects something the organization is trying to improve. Good KPIs are commonly described as **SMART**: Specific, Measurable, Achievable, Relevant, and Time-bound. In healthcare, KPIs span clinical quality (hospital-acquired infection rate, readmission rate), operational efficiency (average length of stay, emergency department wait time, bed turnaround), financial performance (days in accounts receivable, denial rate), and patient experience (HCAHPS scores). The discipline of KPI selection is to choose a small number of meaningful, actionable measures aligned to organizational objectives—rather than overwhelming users with every available metric. A dashboard cluttered with dozens of indicators no one acts on is a common failure mode; a focused set tied to goals is the aim.

> **Key Concept**
>
> An operational report is detailed and transactional, supporting day-to-day work; an analytic dashboard is summarized, visual, and indicator-driven, supporting monitoring and decision-making. KPIs—ideally SMART and aligned to organizational goals—are the measures both are built around.

.33 Visualization Best Practices and Trend Interpretation

How data is displayed determines whether it informs or misleads, so data visualization is a core competency for anyone building reports and dashboards.

The first principle is **choosing the right chart for the message**. Different chart types serve different purposes: a **bar chart** compares discrete categories (infection rates across units); a **line chart** shows change over time (monthly admissions across a year); a **pie chart** shows parts of a whole and is best limited to a few slices because the human eye judges angles poorly; a **scatter plot** shows the relationship between two continuous variables; and a **histogram** shows the distribution of a single variable. Selecting a chart type that does not match the question—using a pie chart for time trends, for instance—confuses the audience.

The second principle is **clarity through simplicity**. The data analyst and educator Edward Tufte popularized the term **chartjunk**—unnecessary decoration, heavy gridlines, distracting backgrounds, gratuitous 3-D effects, and excess ink that adds no information and obscures the message. Best practice strips away clutter so the data itself stands out: clear titles, labeled axes, sensible scales, and the minimum visual elements needed. A related caution is the **truncated y-axis**: starting a bar chart's axis at a value other than zero can exaggerate small differences and mislead viewers, so bar charts should generally begin at zero.

The third principle is **accessibility**. Visualizations must be usable by people with visual impairments, including color blindness, which affects a meaningful share of the population. This means never relying on color alone to convey meaning—pairing color with labels, patterns, or shapes; choosing color-blind-safe palettes; ensuring adequate contrast; and providing text alternatives where appropriate. Accessible design is both an ethical obligation and, in many contexts, a regulatory expectation.

A specialized but important display is the **run chart**, a simple line graph of a measure plotted over time in sequence, usually with a centerline at the median. Run charts are a staple of healthcare quality improvement because they reveal how a process behaves over time and whether an intervention had an effect. Analysts look for non-random patterns—a **shift** (several consecutive points on one side of the median), a **trend** (several consecutive points all increasing or all decreasing), and **runs**—to distinguish genuine change from ordinary variation. A single high or low point is usually just noise; a sustained pattern signals that something real has changed. The more rigorous cousin of the run chart, the **statistical process control (SPC) chart** or control chart, adds calculated control limits to separate **common-cause variation** (the inherent, expected fluctuation of a stable process) from **special-cause variation** (a signal that something unusual has occurred and warrants investigation). For the associate level, the key takeaway is that you do not react to every wiggle in a metric—you look for sustained, non-random patterns before concluding that performance has truly changed.

.34 Data Quality and Governance

Analytics is only as trustworthy as the data beneath it, and poor data quality is among the most common reasons reports mislead. The CAHIMS candidate should know the standard **dimensions of data quality**:

- **Completeness** — the degree to which all required data is present, with no missing values. A patient record lacking a documented allergy field is incomplete.
- **Accuracy** — the degree to which data correctly reflects the real-world fact it represents. A weight recorded as 700 pounds when the patient weighs 170 is inaccurate.
- **Consistency** — the degree to which data agrees with itself across systems and records, with no contradictions. A patient listed as deceased in one system but receiving active orders in another is inconsistent.
- **Timeliness** — the degree to which data is available when needed and reflects the current state. A lab result that posts hours after the clinician needed it fails timeliness.
- **Validity** — the degree to which data conforms to defined formats, ranges, and rules (a date that is actually a valid calendar date; a code that exists in the code set).
- **Uniqueness** — the absence of unintended duplicate records, such as a single patient appearing under two medical record numbers.

These dimensions are interrelated and are the measurable targets of data quality programs. Note the relationship to ETL: the transform stage is where many quality problems are detected and corrected.

Sustaining data quality over time requires **data governance**—the overall framework of policies, roles, standards, and processes that define how an organization manages its data assets, who is accountable, and how decisions about data are made. Governance answers questions such as: Who owns each data element? How are definitions agreed upon? Who may access what, and under what controls? A central role in this framework is the **data steward**, an individual—often a subject-matter expert in a clinical or operational area—responsible for the quality, definition, and appropriate use of specific data within their domain. Data stewardship is the operational, hands-on side of governance: stewards adjudicate definitions, monitor quality, and serve as the accountable point of contact for their data.

A foundational governance artifact is the **data dictionary**—a centralized reference that documents each data element: its name, definition, data type, allowed values or format, source, and relationships. The data dictionary ensures that everyone in the organization means the same thing by a term like "admission" or "active patient," which is essential because inconsistent definitions are a frequent cause of conflicting reports. When two dashboards show different readmission rates, the cause is often that each used a different, undocumented definition—precisely the problem a data dictionary prevents. Related governance practices include managing **master data** (such as a master patient index that resolves duplicate patient identities) and maintaining **metadata**, the descriptive "data about data" that the data dictionary captures.

For the candidate, the unifying theme is that analytics is not merely a technical exercise in charts and queries. It rests on a disciplined foundation of integrated, high-quality data, governed by clear policies and stewarded by accountable people, and translated into focused indicators and honest visualizations. Get the foundation right and the climb from data to wisdom becomes possible; neglect it and even sophisticated dashboards will mislead.

> **Exam Tip**
>
> Know the data quality dimensions cold—completeness, accuracy, consistency, timeliness, validity, uniqueness—and remember that the **data dictionary** standardizes element definitions while the **data steward** is the accountable person for data quality within a domain. Scenario questions frequently test whether you can match a problem ("two reports disagree on a metric") to its remedy ("a shared definition in the data dictionary").

.35 Chapter 9 Review Questions

Q1. A hospital quality team builds a model that uses historical data to estimate each admitted patient's probability of being readmitted within 30 days. Which type of analytics does this represent?
A) Descriptive analytics
B) Diagnostic analytics
C) Predictive analytics
D) Prescriptive analytics

Answer: C — Estimating the probability of a future event ("What is likely to happen?") from historical data is predictive analytics. Descriptive summarizes what already happened, diagnostic explains why it happened, and prescriptive recommends a specific action to take.

Q2. In a relational database, an "Encounters" table includes a column containing patient IDs that correspond to the unique identifier in the "Patients" table. What is this patient ID column called within the Encounters table?
A) Primary key
B) Foreign key
C) Composite index
D) Metadata field

Answer: B — A foreign key is a column in one table that references the primary key of another table, establishing the relationship between them. The unique identifier in the Patients table is the primary key; its appearance in Encounters as a link makes it a foreign key there.

Q3. A healthcare organization extracts data from its EHR, lab, and billing systems; cleans and standardizes it so codes and formats are consistent; and writes it into a central enterprise data warehouse for analysis. The cleaning-and-standardizing step is part of which process?
A) Normalization
B) The transform stage of ETL
C) A SQL JOIN
D) Data stewardship

Answer: B — Extract, Transform, Load (ETL) moves data into a warehouse; the transform stage is where data is cleaned, standardized, deduplicated, and mapped to common formats before loading. Normalization is a database design principle, a JOIN combines tables in a query, and stewardship is a governance role.

Q4. A dashboard designer wants to display monthly emergency department patient volume over the past twelve months so leaders can spot trends. Which chart type and design choice are most appropriate?
A) A pie chart, because it shows parts of a whole
B) A line chart with a y-axis starting at zero and minimal chartjunk
C) A 3-D bar chart with decorative background images for visual appeal
D) A scatter plot of volume against patient age

Answer: B — A line chart is the correct choice for showing change in a single measure over time. Best practice keeps the design clean (minimal chartjunk) and avoids misleading scales. A pie chart shows composition, not trends; 3-D effects and decoration are chartjunk; and a scatter plot addresses relationships between two variables, not a time trend.

Q5. Two dashboards in the same hospital report different 30-day readmission rates for the same period because each was built using a different, undocumented definition of "readmission." Which governance artifact most directly prevents this problem?
A) A data warehouse
B) A run chart
C) A data dictionary
D) A primary key

Answer: C — A data dictionary standardizes the definition, data type, allowed values, and source of each data element, ensuring everyone means the same thing by a term like "readmission." A data warehouse stores integrated data but does not by itself define terms; a run chart displays a measure over time; and a primary key uniquely identifies database rows.

Emerging Technologies — AI, Telehealth, Cloud, and Cybersecurity Operations

Exam Weight: Approximately 10–14 percent (Emerging Technology and Security)

.36 Learning Objectives

After completing this chapter, the candidate will be able to:

- Describe foundational concepts of artificial intelligence and machine learning in healthcare, including supervised and unsupervised approaches, common clinical and administrative use cases, the FDA Software as a Medical Device framework, and the importance of monitoring for algorithmic bias.
- Explain how generative artificial intelligence and large language models are applied in clinical and administrative settings, and identify their characteristic risks.
- Differentiate among telehealth and virtual care modalities — synchronous, asynchronous (store-and-forward), and remote patient monitoring — and the operational and quality considerations each raises.
- Compare cloud computing service models (IaaS, PaaS, SaaS) and deployment models (public, private, hybrid), and apply the shared-responsibility model to healthcare environments.
- Summarize core cybersecurity operations concepts — the CIA triad, defense-in-depth, common threats, multi-factor authentication, least privilege, security awareness training, incident response, and the role of the HHS 405(d) Health Industry Cybersecurity Practices.

.37 Artificial Intelligence and Machine Learning Foundations

Artificial intelligence (AI) is a broad field concerned with building computer systems that perform tasks normally requiring human intelligence, such as recognizing patterns, making predictions, and interpreting language. **Machine learning (ML)** is the subfield of AI most relevant to healthcare today. Rather than following explicitly programmed rules, a machine learning system *learns* statistical patterns from data and applies those patterns to new, unseen cases. The associate-level professional is not expected to build models, but is expected to understand the vocabulary, the common uses, and the governance obligations.

Machine learning approaches fall into a few major categories. In **supervised learning**, the model is trained on labeled examples — data in which the correct answer is already known. A model trained to flag diabetic retinopathy, for instance, learns from thousands of retinal images that clinicians have already labeled as showing disease or not showing disease. The model's goal is to generalize from those labeled examples so it can classify new images. Supervised learning underlies most clinical prediction and image-classification tools. In **unsupervised learning**, the model receives data without labels and is asked to find structure on its own — grouping similar patients into clusters, for example, or detecting unusual records that may represent fraud or data-quality problems. A third family, **reinforcement learning**, in which a system learns through trial-and-error feedback, appears in research settings such as treatment-sequencing simulations but is less common in deployed healthcare products.

Three clinical use cases recur often enough that the associate should know them. The first is **medical imaging**: ML models assist radiologists, pathologists, and ophthalmologists by detecting and triaging findings on X-rays, CT scans, mammograms, and digital pathology slides. These tools typically act as a "second reader" or triage aid rather than a replacement for the clinician. The second is **risk prediction**: models estimate the likelihood of a future event — sepsis, hospital readmission, patient deterioration, or no-show appointments — so that care teams can intervene early. The third, and the fastest-growing in 2026, is **ambient clinical documentation**: AI systems listen to the clinician-patient conversation and automatically draft a clinical note, reducing the documentation burden that drives clinician burnout.

> **Key Concept**
> Supervised learning uses *labeled* data to predict a known outcome; unsupervised learning finds structure in *unlabeled* data. If the exam describes a model trained on images already marked "disease" or "no disease," that is supervised learning.

Because some AI tools influence diagnosis or treatment, they may be regulated as medical devices. The **U.S. Food and Drug Administration (FDA)** uses the framework of **Software as a Medical Device (SaMD)** — software intended for one or more medical purposes that performs those purposes without being part of a hardware device. Whether a particular AI product requires FDA review depends on its intended use and the risk it poses to patients; a tool that diagnoses disease autonomously faces far more scrutiny than one that merely schedules appointments. The FDA has cleared or authorized a large and growing number of AI- and ML-enabled medical devices, and it has developed a **Predetermined Change Control Plan** approach to address a unique property of machine learning: these models can be retrained and updated over time. The associate should understand the principle — that adaptive software requires a plan for how it will change safely — rather than memorize regulatory minutiae.

A central governance obligation for any deployed model is the management of **algorithmic bias.** A model learns whatever patterns exist in its training data, including patterns that reflect historical inequities. If a model is trained predominantly on data from one population, it may perform poorly for under-represented groups, producing less accurate predictions for them. A well-documented example involved a risk-stratification algorithm that used historical healthcare spending as a proxy for health need; because less money had historically been spent on certain patients, the model systematically underestimated their needs. Bias of this kind is rarely intentional, which is precisely why **ongoing monitoring** is required. Organizations must validate models on their own patient populations before deployment, watch for performance drift after deployment, and establish governance committees that review AI tools across their lifecycle. The lesson for the associate is durable: an AI system is never "finished" at go-live — it must be continuously measured against real-world outcomes.

.38 Generative AI and Large Language Models

A distinct and rapidly maturing branch of AI is **generative AI**, which produces new content — text, images, audio, or code — rather than simply classifying existing data. The most consequential generative technology in healthcare is the **large language model (LLM)**, a model trained on vast quantities of text that can understand and generate human-like language. LLMs power the ambient documentation tools mentioned earlier, draft patient-friendly summaries of clinical results, answer staff questions about policies, assist with prior-authorization letters and coding, and respond to routine patient messages in the patient portal under clinician supervision.

The benefits are real, but so are the risks, and the associate must be able to name them. The most important is **hallucination** — the tendency of an LLM to generate fluent, confident text that is factually incorrect or entirely fabricated. Because the output reads plausibly, a clinician or staff member who does not verify it may act on false information. A second risk is **protected health information (PHI) exposure**: entering patient data into a public, consumer-grade AI service may transmit that data outside the organization's control and violate HIPAA. Healthcare organizations therefore require a **Business Associate Agreement (BAA)** before any AI vendor may process PHI. Additional risks include **bias** carried from training data, lack of **transparency** (the difficulty of explaining why a model produced a given output), and **data privacy** concerns about how prompts are retained and reused.

The governance response is captured in the principle of **human oversight**, sometimes phrased as keeping a "human in the loop." Generative AI output that affects care or compliance should be reviewed and approved by a qualified person before it is finalized. Organizations are also adopting **responsible AI** governance frameworks — guidance such as the **NIST AI Risk Management Framework** provides a structured way to manage AI risk, and many provider organizations have stood up internal AI governance committees to vet tools before adoption. For the CAHIMS candidate, the essential takeaway is that generative AI is a powerful productivity tool whose outputs must be verified, whose access to PHI must be governed by a BAA, and whose use must be supervised by accountable humans.

.39 Telehealth and Virtual Care Modalities

Telehealth is the use of telecommunications and information technology to deliver health-related services at a distance. (The narrower term **telemedicine** usually refers specifically to remote clinical care, while telehealth also encompasses remote education and administrative services.) Adoption accelerated sharply during the COVID-19 public health emergency and, although utilization has moderated since, virtual care has become a permanent and expected modality. The associate should be able to distinguish the three principal modalities.

Synchronous telehealth is real-time, two-way interaction between a patient and a provider, most commonly a live video visit, though it can also be audio-only. The defining feature is simultaneity: both parties are present at the same time, as in a conventional office encounter conducted over video. **Asynchronous telehealth**, often called **store-and-forward**, does not require both parties to participate at once. Clinical information — images, messages, or recorded data — is captured, stored, and then transmitted to a provider who reviews it later and responds. Teledermatology, in which a photograph of a skin lesion is sent to a specialist for review, and the review of retinal images in teleophthalmology are classic store-and-forward examples. **Remote patient monitoring (RPM)** uses connected devices — blood pressure cuffs, glucometers, pulse oximeters, weight scales, and wearables — to collect physiological data from a patient at home and transmit it to the care team for review and intervention. RPM is especially valuable for managing chronic conditions such as hypertension, diabetes, and heart failure, where trends over time matter more than a single in-office reading.

> **Exam Tip**
>
> Match the modality to the timing. *Synchronous* = real-time (live video). *Asynchronous / store-and-forward* = capture now, review later (teledermatology photo). *Remote patient monitoring* = connected home devices streaming physiological data to the care team.

Several operational and quality considerations apply across modalities. **Licensure and reimbursement** are jurisdiction-dependent: providers generally must be licensed where the patient is located, and coverage policies for telehealth — including which services qualify and whether audio-only visits are reimbursed — vary by payer and continue to evolve. **Technology access and the digital divide** affect equity, because patients without reliable broadband, a suitable device, or digital literacy may be unable to participate, which can widen rather than narrow disparities. **Privacy and security** obligations apply fully to virtual care: the platform must be HIPAA-compliant, the connection encrypted, and patient identity verified. **Workflow integration** matters because telehealth visits and RPM data must flow into the EHR so the record remains complete and the data is actionable. Finally, **clinical appropriateness** governs which conditions can safely be managed remotely versus which require an in-person examination. The associate's role is frequently to support these operational requirements — confirming platform compliance, integrating data into the EHR, and helping ensure equitable access.

.40 Cloud Computing in Healthcare

Healthcare organizations increasingly run their applications and store their data in the **cloud** rather than in on-premises data centers. **Cloud computing** is the on-demand delivery of computing resources — servers, storage, databases, software — over the internet, typically paid for as a metered service. The appeal is **scalability** (resources expand and contract with demand), reduced **capital expenditure** (no large up-front hardware purchases), and **reliability** through professionally managed infrastructure. The associate should know the standard service and deployment models, which the **National Institute of Standards and Technology (NIST)** defines.

There are three core **service models. Infrastructure as a Service (IaaS)** provides fundamental computing building blocks — virtual servers, storage, and networking — which the customer configures and manages. The customer controls the operating system and applications; the provider manages the underlying physical infrastructure. **Platform as a Service (PaaS)** adds a managed development and deployment platform on top of the infrastructure, so developers can build and run applications without managing the servers or operating systems beneath them. **Software as a Service (SaaS)** delivers a complete, ready-to-use application over the internet; the customer simply uses the software through a browser while the provider manages everything underneath. Most healthcare staff interact daily with SaaS — a cloud-hosted EHR, a web-based scheduling tool, or an email platform are familiar examples.

A useful way to remember the distinction is how much the customer manages: with IaaS the customer manages the most (everything above the virtual hardware); with PaaS, only the applications and data; with SaaS, the least, often just user accounts and configuration settings.

Deployment models describe where the cloud resources live and who can access them. A **public cloud** is owned and operated by a third-party provider and shared among many customers (tenants), offering the greatest scale and lowest cost. A **private cloud** is dedicated to a single organization, providing more control and isolation — sometimes preferred for highly sensitive workloads. A **hybrid cloud** combines public and private (and possibly on-premises) environments so that workloads can be placed where they best fit; an organization might keep its most sensitive data in a private environment while bursting less-sensitive analytics into the public cloud. Many healthcare organizations operate hybrid environments for exactly this reason.

> **Key Concept**
>
> The **shared-responsibility model** divides security duties between the cloud provider and the customer. The provider secures the cloud *infrastructure* ("security *of* the cloud"); the customer secures what it puts *in* the cloud ("security *in* the cloud") — its data, access controls, and configurations. The model shifts depending on the service tier, but the customer is *never* fully relieved of responsibility.

The **shared-responsibility model** deserves special attention because it is a frequent source of real-world breaches and a likely exam topic. Moving to the cloud does not transfer all security responsibility to the vendor. Under IaaS the customer is responsible for securing the operating system, applications, and data; under SaaS the provider handles more of the stack, but the customer remains responsible for managing user access, configuring the application securely, and protecting its data. Misconfigured cloud storage left open to the public internet is one of the most common causes of healthcare data exposure — a failure of customer responsibility, not provider failure. Regardless of service model, the healthcare customer remains the **HIPAA-covered entity** accountable for protecting PHI, and it must execute a **Business Associate Agreement** with any cloud vendor that stores or processes that data.

.41 Interoperability Advances

Emerging technologies deliver value only when systems can exchange data, which makes **interoperability** a recurring theme. Chapter coverage elsewhere in this guide introduced the foundational standards; here the focus is on the advances shaping 2026.

The leading modern standard is **HL7 FHIR — Fast Healthcare Interoperability Resources**. FHIR organizes health data into modular, discrete units called **resources** (for example, Patient, Observation, Medication, Encounter) and exchanges them using familiar web technologies such as **RESTful APIs** and standard data formats. This web-friendly design makes FHIR easier to implement than older message-based standards and has made it the backbone of the modern API economy in health IT, including the app interfaces patients use to access their own records. The associate should know that FHIR is **resource-based and API-driven**, which is what distinguishes it from earlier HL7 messaging.

Two regulatory and infrastructure advances build on FHIR. The **United States Core Data for Interoperability (USCDI)** is a standardized set of data classes and data elements — defined and periodically expanded by the federal government — that must be available for nationwide electronic exchange. USCDI establishes a common baseline so that certified systems all share at least a core vocabulary of patient information. The **Trusted Exchange Framework and Common Agreement (TEFCA)** establishes a nationwide "network of networks" for health information exchange, governed by a single common agreement. Within TEFCA, **Qualified Health Information Networks (QHINs)** are the designated organizations that connect to one another and serve as the on-ramps through which participants exchange data across the country. TEFCA became operational, with QHINs exchanging data, and continues to expand its scope toward broader, FHIR-based exchange. For the associate, the high-level relationship is what matters: **USCDI** defines *what* data is shared, **FHIR** increasingly defines *how* it is technically exchanged, and **TEFCA/QHINs** provide the nationwide *governance and connectivity* that lets organizations exchange that data under common rules.

.42 Cybersecurity Operations

Healthcare is among the most-targeted sectors for cyberattack because patient data is valuable and because disruptions to care create urgent pressure to pay. Every associate, regardless of role, shares responsibility for security. The conceptual foundation is the **CIA triad**, the three properties a security program protects: **Confidentiality** (information is accessible only to those authorized to see it), **Integrity** (information is accurate and has not been improperly altered), and **Availability** (information and systems are accessible to authorized users when needed). A ransomware attack that locks clinicians out of the EHR is fundamentally an *availability* failure; an unauthorized record disclosure is a *confidentiality* failure; tampering with a lab result is an *integrity* failure.

Security programs implement **defense-in-depth** — the layering of multiple, independent controls so that the failure of any single control does not result in compromise. Layers span physical controls (locked facilities), technical controls (firewalls, encryption, endpoint protection), and administrative controls (policies and training). No single safeguard is sufficient on its own.

The associate should recognize the most common threats. **Phishing** is a social-engineering attack in which an attacker sends fraudulent communications, usually email, designed to trick a recipient into revealing credentials, clicking a malicious link, or opening an infected attachment; it remains the leading initial entry point for healthcare breaches. **Ransomware** is malicious software that encrypts an organization's data and demands payment for its release; in healthcare it can halt clinical operations and force diversion of patients, making it a patient-safety issue as much as a data issue. Other threats include **malware** generally, **insider threats** (whether malicious or accidental), and **business email compromise**, in which attackers impersonate executives or vendors to redirect payments.

> **Exam Tip**
>
> Tie each threat or control back to the **CIA triad** and remember the human element. **Phishing** is the most common *entry point*; **ransomware** primarily attacks *availability*; **multi-factor authentication** defends against stolen passwords; and **security awareness training** addresses the reality that people, not technology, are the most frequently exploited weakness.

Several specific controls recur on the exam. **Multi-factor authentication (MFA)** requires two or more independent forms of verification — typically something you *know* (a password) plus something you *have* (a phone or token) or something you *are* (a fingerprint). MFA dramatically reduces the impact of stolen passwords and is now a baseline expectation. The **principle of least privilege** holds that each user, system, or process should be granted only the minimum access necessary to perform its function and no more, which limits the damage a compromised account can do. **Security awareness training** educates the workforce to recognize phishing and follow good security hygiene; because people are the most frequently exploited vector, regular training — including simulated phishing exercises — is one of the highest-value investments an organization can make. **Encryption** protects data both *at rest* (stored) and *in transit* (moving across networks) so that intercepted or stolen data remains unreadable.

When prevention fails, **incident response** governs how the organization reacts. A standard incident response lifecycle, reflecting widely used NIST guidance, includes **preparation** (having a plan, tools, and trained team in place), **detection and analysis** (identifying that an incident has occurred and assessing its scope), **containment, eradication, and recovery** (isolating affected systems, removing the threat, and restoring operations from clean backups), and **post-incident activity** (capturing lessons learned to improve future defenses). For healthcare specifically, incident response intersects with regulatory duties: a breach of unsecured PHI triggers **HIPAA Breach Notification Rule** obligations to notify affected individuals, the U.S. Department of Health and Human Services (HHS), and in larger breaches the media, within defined timeframes. The associate need not manage an incident, but should understand the phases and know that breach notification is a legal requirement, not an option.

Healthcare-specific guidance comes from the **HHS 405(d) Program** and its flagship publication, **Health Industry Cybersecurity Practices (HICP)**. Created under Section 405(d) of the Cybersecurity Act of 2015 through a public-private partnership, the 405(d) Program provides voluntary, consensus-based practices tailored to the sector. HICP identifies the leading threats facing healthcare and recommends practical mitigations scaled to organizations of different sizes, helping smaller practices and large health systems alike prioritize their defenses. Recognizing these practices can also be advantageous when regulators assess an organization's security posture after an incident. For the CAHIMS candidate, the key fact is that **405(d) / HICP** is the principal *healthcare-specific* cybersecurity guidance, distinct from broader frameworks such as the **NIST Cybersecurity Framework** that apply across all industries.

.43 IoT and Medical Device Security

A final and increasingly urgent dimension of healthcare cybersecurity is the security of connected devices. The **Internet of Things (IoT)** refers to the growing population of network-connected physical devices, and in healthcare the relevant subset is the **Internet of Medical Things (IoMT)** — infusion pumps, patient monitors, imaging systems, smart beds, and a wide range of other connected clinical equipment. These devices expand the **attack surface** of the organization: each one is a potential entry point, and many are difficult to secure for reasons the associate should understand.

Medical devices frequently run **legacy or unpatchable software**, sometimes because the manufacturer no longer supports the operating system or because patching requires regulatory re-validation that delays updates. Many devices ship with **default passwords** that are never changed, and some cannot be taken offline for maintenance because they are in continuous clinical use. The consequences of compromise are uniquely serious: a successful attack on a connected medical device can threaten not only data but **patient safety** directly.

The mitigation strategies are practical and management-oriented. **Asset inventory** is the foundation — an organization cannot protect devices it does not know it has, so a complete inventory of connected medical devices is the first step. **Network segmentation** isolates medical devices on separate network zones so that a compromise in one area cannot easily spread to clinical systems. **Vulnerability management** tracks known weaknesses and applies vendor patches as they become available. Robust **vendor and procurement practices** push security requirements upstream, and the **Software Bill of Materials (SBOM)** — a formal list of the software components inside a device — helps organizations respond to vulnerabilities in those components. The FDA now expects manufacturers to address cybersecurity throughout a device's lifecycle, including providing SBOMs and a plan for handling discovered vulnerabilities. The associate's likely contribution is operational: supporting the device inventory, helping enforce segmentation, and coordinating with vendors and the security team. The unifying principle of this chapter holds here as well — emerging technology delivers value only when it is governed, monitored, and secured throughout its lifecycle, with patient safety and data protection as the constant priorities.

.44 Chapter 10 Review Questions

Q1. A health system trains a model using thousands of chest X-ray images that radiologists have already labeled as either "pneumonia" or "no pneumonia," so the model can classify new images. Which machine learning approach does this describe?

A) Unsupervised learning
B) Supervised learning
C) Reinforcement learning
D) Generative learning

Answer: B — The model learns from *labeled* examples (each image is marked with the known correct outcome) in order to predict that outcome on new cases. That is the defining characteristic of supervised learning. Unsupervised learning works with unlabeled data to find structure, and reinforcement learning learns through trial-and-error feedback.

Q2. A clinic uses a public, consumer-grade generative AI chatbot to draft patient message responses, and a staff member pastes a patient's name and diagnosis into it. What is the most significant concern with this practice?

A) The chatbot may respond too slowly for clinical workflow
B) Protected health information may be exposed to an external service without a Business Associate Agreement
C) Generative AI cannot produce grammatically correct text
D) The chatbot will automatically delete the patient record

Answer: B — Entering PHI into a public AI service transmits that data outside the organization's control. HIPAA requires a Business Associate Agreement with any vendor that processes PHI, and consumer-grade tools typically lack one, creating a privacy and compliance violation. (Hallucination is also a real generative-AI risk, but the question specifically concerns exposing patient identifiers to an outside service.)

Q3. A patient photographs a suspicious skin lesion and sends the image through a portal to a dermatologist, who reviews it several hours later and replies with an assessment. Which telehealth modality is this?

A) Synchronous telehealth
B) Remote patient monitoring

C) Asynchronous (store-and-forward) telehealth
D) Inpatient telemetry

Answer: C — The information is captured, stored, and then reviewed later by the provider, who is not present at the same time as the patient. That capture-now/review-later pattern defines asynchronous, or store-and-forward, telehealth — teledermatology is a classic example. Synchronous care is real-time, and remote patient monitoring streams data from connected home devices.

Q4. A hospital uses a public cloud provider to host a database of patient information. A staff member misconfigures the storage so it is openly accessible on the internet, resulting in a data exposure. Under the shared-responsibility model, who bears responsibility for this misconfiguration?

A) The cloud provider, because it owns the infrastructure
B) The hospital, because securing its data and configurations in the cloud is the customer's responsibility
C) No one, because cloud data is automatically secured
D) The HHS 405(d) Program

Answer: B — Under the shared-responsibility model, the provider secures the cloud infrastructure ("security *of* the cloud"), but the customer is responsible for what it places in the cloud ("security *in* the cloud") — including its data and configuration settings. Misconfigured, publicly exposed storage is a customer responsibility, and the hospital remains the HIPAA-covered entity accountable for the PHI.

Q5. A small physician practice wants healthcare-specific, voluntary guidance for prioritizing defenses against the most common cyber threats facing the industry. Which resource is designed specifically for this purpose?

A) The HHS 405(d) Health Industry Cybersecurity Practices (HICP)
B) The HL7 FHIR specification
C) The United States Core Data for Interoperability (USCDI)
D) The Predetermined Change Control Plan

Answer: A — The HHS 405(d) Program's Health Industry Cybersecurity Practices (HICP) provides voluntary, consensus-based, *healthcare-specific* guidance scaled to organizations of different sizes, helping them prioritize mitigations for the sector's leading threats. FHIR and USCDI are interoperability standards, and the Predetermined Change Control Plan is an FDA concept for adaptive AI/ML medical devices.

.45 Practice Examination Two

This is the second of two full-length practice examinations and approximates the content proportions of the CAHIMS exam blueprint, with the heaviest weighting on the Technology Environment, Systems, and Privacy and Security domains and lighter coverage of the Healthcare Environment and Administration/Leadership domains. Budget approximately 1.5 minutes per item (about 75 minutes for the complete 50-question exam). Items are written at entry level with some application stems; after scoring, read each rationale in full so that you reinforce the underlying concept and the reasoning behind the distractors rather than memorizing only the correct letter.

Q1. During your first week as a clinical informatics associate, a project lead asks you to explain why the hospital exchanges patient data using a widely recognized messaging standard instead of a vendor's proprietary format. The lead notes that the laboratory, pharmacy, and registration systems all need to share data even though they were built by different companies, and asks which body actually writes and maintains the HL7 Version 2.x and FHIR standards that make this possible. Which organization is responsible for developing the HL7 family of interoperability standards?

A) The Office of the National Coordinator for Health IT (ONC)
B) Health Level Seven International
C) The Centers for Medicare & Medicaid Services (CMS)
D) The National Institute of Standards and Technology (NIST)

Answer: B — Health Level Seven International (HL7) is the volunteer-driven, ANSI-accredited standards development organization that authors and maintains HL7 V2.x messaging, the V3 and Clinical Document Architecture (CDA) family, and FHIR. The "Level Seven" in its name references the application layer (Layer 7) of the OSI networking model, reflecting that these are application-level data standards. ONC and CMS are federal agencies that may require, incentivize, or certify the use of such standards through regulation and programs, but they do not author the clinical messaging standards themselves. NIST publishes cybersecurity frameworks and technical guidance rather than clinical interoperability standards, so knowing who owns a standard helps you direct technical questions to the correct authority and read implementation guides correctly. Key concept: HL7 is a standards body, while ONC and CMS are regulators that may mandate the use of HL7's standards but do not author them.

Q2. A vendor representative tells your team that their new patient-engagement app exchanges data "the modern way," using web technologies rather than the older pipe-delimited messages your interface team is used to. The representative explains that developers can call an endpoint and retrieve discrete pieces of a patient's record on demand, much like any contemporary web application. The representative is describing FHIR (Fast Healthcare Interoperability Resources). Which statement best captures a core technical characteristic of FHIR that distinguishes it from legacy HL7 Version 2 messaging?

A) It relies exclusively on flat-file batch transfers exchanged on a nightly schedule
B) It can only transmit radiology imaging studies in DICOM format
C) It is built on modern web standards such as RESTful APIs and represents data as modular resources serialized in JSON or XML
D) It eliminates the need for any authentication because all exchanged data is automatically de-identified

Answer: C — FHIR organizes health data into modular "resources" — for example, Patient, Observation, MedicationRequest, and AllergyIntolerance — that are exchanged through RESTful web APIs and commonly serialized as JSON or XML. This web-friendly, granular design is precisely what separates it from older HL7 V2 messages that use segments and pipe-delimited fields, and it is why third-party app developers can build against a FHIR endpoint much as they would against any modern web service. FHIR does not de-identify data and absolutely still requires strong authentication and authorization, frequently implemented with OAuth 2.0 and the SMART on FHIR profile. Its modularity allows applications to request only the specific resources they need, and ONC's certification criteria require certified EHRs to expose a standardized FHIR-based API for patient and population data access. Key concept: FHIR's use of REST plus JSON/XML resources is the defining contrast with the older segment-and-pipe structure of HL7 V2.

Q3. A small clinic that is joining a regional health information exchange worries that each EHR vendor defines its core patient data fields differently, which has made past data exchange unreliable and inconsistent. The clinic's IT manager asks whether there is a single, vendor-neutral list that every certified EHR must be able to share, so that demographics, problems, medications, allergies, and lab results all arrive in a predictable form. You explain that ONC publishes exactly such a standardized minimum set of data classes and elements. Which standard defines that minimum, vendor-neutral set?

A) USCDI (United States Core Data for Interoperability)
B) ICD-10-CM
C) NCPDP SCRIPT
D) X12 837

Answer: A — The United States Core Data for Interoperability (USCDI) is the ONC-maintained, standardized set of health data classes and constituent data elements — such as patient demographics, problems, medications, allergies, immunizations, clinical notes, and laboratory results — required for nationwide interoperable exchange. USCDI is expanded over time through a public, predictable versioning process (USCDI v1, v2, v3, and beyond), so the floor of shareable data grows steadily and vendors can plan for it. It is important to recognize that USCDI defines *what* data must be shareable, not *how* it travels; the transport is handled by standards such as FHIR. ICD-10-CM is a diagnosis code set, NCPDP SCRIPT governs electronic prescribing transactions, and X12 837 is the standard format for submitting healthcare claims — none of these defines the cross-vendor minimum data set. Key concept: USCDI is a content standard (the data), not a transport, code, or transaction standard.

Q4. Your compliance officer reminds the team that the HIPAA Privacy Rule protects "individually identifiable health information" held or transmitted by covered entities and business associates. You are reviewing four data sets to determine which one falls outside the definition of protected health information (PHI). Which of the following would NOT, by itself, be considered PHI?

A) A patient's full name linked to a specific diagnosis
B) A medical record number associated with a particular treatment date
C) A patient's home address combined with their laboratory results
D) A data set that has been de-identified by removing all 18 identifiers under the Safe Harbor method

Answer: D — Information that has been properly de-identified — either by removing all 18 Safe Harbor identifiers (including names, geographic subdivisions smaller than a state, all elements of dates except year, and contact and device identifiers) or through the expert determination method — is no longer individually identifiable and therefore is not PHI, falling outside the Privacy Rule's use and disclosure restrictions. Each of the other options links identifying information (a name, a medical record number, or a home address) to health information, which squarely meets the definition of PHI. Understanding the de-identification boundary is essential because de-identified data can be used for research, analytics, and quality improvement with far fewer restrictions. Note that re-identifying such data, or creating a code that allows re-identification, can pull the information back under the Privacy Rule. Key concept: removing the 18 Safe Harbor identifiers (or expert determination) is what converts PHI into non-PHI de-identified data.

Q5. The HIPAA Security Rule organizes its required and addressable specifications into three categories of safeguards. In a single review, your team implements role-based access controls in the EHR and also conducts the organization's annual formal risk analysis. These two activities map, respectively, to which categories of safeguards?

A) Physical safeguards and Organizational requirements
B) Technical safeguards and Administrative safeguards
C) Administrative safeguards and Physical safeguards
D) Technical safeguards and Physical safeguards

Answer: B — Access controls that restrict system access according to a user's role are Technical safeguards because they are implemented within the information system itself, alongside other technical controls such as audit controls, integrity controls, and transmission security. The formal, periodic risk analysis and ongoing risk management process is an Administrative safeguard — a policy-and-process activity that drives the organization's overall security program and is widely considered its foundation. Physical safeguards, by contrast, address facility access controls, workstation use and security, and device and media controls. The Security Rule's three safeguard categories are Administrative, Physical, and Technical, and many associates find it useful to remember that "risk analysis is administrative" because it is the planning activity from which the other controls flow. Key concept: controls built into the system are Technical, policies and processes are Administrative, and facility and device protections are Physical.

Q6. A nurse on a pilot unit enters a medication order directly into the EHR using a structured ordering screen, rather than writing the order on paper for a unit clerk to later transcribe into the system. Your director explains that this capability is one of the most important patient-safety functions in a modern EHR because it removes illegible handwriting and the transcription step where errors historically crept in, and that national patient-safety programs have long encouraged its adoption. What is this functionality called?

A) Clinical decision support (CDS)
B) Health information exchange (HIE)
C) Computerized provider order entry (CPOE)
D) Master patient index (MPI)

Answer: C — Computerized provider order entry (CPOE) allows authorized clinicians to enter orders for medications, laboratory tests, and imaging directly into the system, eliminating illegible handwriting and the error-prone manual transcription step that paper orders required. CPOE is one of the most studied patient-safety functions in health IT and is frequently paired with clinical decision support, which supplies the alerts and guidance, but the order-entry capability itself is CPOE. Health information exchange (HIE) moves data between separate organizations, and the master patient index (MPI) manages and reconciles patient identity across systems. Distinguishing CPOE (entering orders) from CDS (advising on those orders) is a common exam point. Key concept: CPOE is the act of entering the order electronically; the alerts that fire during entry are CDS.

Q7. A physician using CPOE places an order for a new antibiotic, and the EHR immediately displays a warning that the drug may interact dangerously with a medication the patient is already taking. Your team is asked to categorize the type of functionality that produced this alert. This interaction warning is an example of:

A) A drug-drug interaction check provided by clinical decision support
B) A revenue cycle charge edit
C) A FHIR Bulk Data export job
D) An interface engine message acknowledgment

Answer: A — Drug-drug interaction alerts, drug-allergy warnings, dosing guidance, duplicate-therapy checks, and preventive-care reminders are classic forms of clinical decision support (CDS), which delivers patient-specific knowledge at the point of care to improve safety and quality. The other options are unrelated: a revenue cycle edit catches billing or coding problems, a FHIR Bulk Data export moves large population-level data sets for analytics, and an interface acknowledgment (an HL7 ACK message) merely confirms message receipt between systems. Well-tuned CDS reduces preventable harm, but excessive or poorly targeted alerts can cause "alert fatigue," in which clinicians begin to override or ignore warnings — a key reason CDS must be carefully governed and tuned over time. Key concept: any patient-specific knowledge delivered at the point of care to guide a decision is clinical decision support.

Q8. A project manager is documenting precisely what an EHR optimization project will and will not deliver, including features that are explicitly excluded from this phase. A new associate asks why this careful boundary-setting matters. Documenting these boundaries primarily helps the team prevent:

A) Scope creep
B) Data normalization
C) Two-factor authentication
D) Network latency

Answer: A — A clearly written scope statement that lists deliverables and explicit exclusions is the principal control against scope creep — the uncontrolled, often informal expansion of project work beyond what was agreed and resourced. When boundaries are vague, stakeholders add "just one more feature" requests that quietly erode the schedule, budget, and quality. Data normalization, two-factor authentication, and network latency are technical concerns unrelated to defining project boundaries. Any legitimate change to an agreed scope should flow through a formal change control process so the impact on cost and timeline is evaluated and approved rather than absorbed silently. Key concept: a documented scope (deliverables plus exclusions) is the primary defense against uncontrolled scope creep, and changes to it should always be evaluated through formal change control rather than accepted informally on the spot.

Q9. Early in a new clinical-system initiative, before any detailed planning or scheduling has been done, the steering committee signs a single document that formally authorizes the project to begin, names the project manager and gives that person authority to use organizational resources, and lists the project's high-level objectives and business justification. Everyone agrees this document is the reference point that legitimizes the effort and the project manager's role. In standard project management practice, what is this document called?

A) Work breakdown structure
B) Risk register
C) Project charter
D) Gantt chart

Answer: C — The project charter is the document that formally authorizes a project's existence, names the project manager and confers authority to apply organizational resources, and states the high-level objectives, business case, and key stakeholders. It is typically the first formal deliverable produced during project initiation and serves as the reference point for whether subsequent work is in scope. The work breakdown structure decomposes the total work into smaller, manageable packages; the risk register catalogs, scores, and tracks risks along with response plans; and a Gantt chart visualizes the schedule as horizontal bars across a timeline. Confusing the charter (authorization) with planning artifacts like the WBS or schedule is a common entry-level error. Key concept: the charter authorizes the project and empowers the project manager; planning documents come afterward.

Q10. A development team is replacing the laboratory information system. Before any screens are designed or code is written, the analysts meet with lab staff to document exactly what the new system must do, including required interfaces to instruments, reporting capabilities, and turnaround-time rules. Within the Systems Development Life Cycle (SDLC), this activity occurs in which phase?

A) Implementation
B) Requirements analysis
C) Maintenance
D) Disposal

Answer: B — Gathering, clarifying, and documenting functional and technical requirements is the core of the requirements analysis (analysis) phase, which precedes design, development, testing, and implementation in the Systems Development Life Cycle. Capturing complete and accurate requirements early is the most cost-effective time to correct misunderstandings, because the cost of fixing a defect rises sharply at each later phase — a problem caught in analysis is far cheaper to resolve than one discovered after go-live. Implementation is the go-live and deployment phase, maintenance keeps the system running and patched afterward, and disposal retires the system at end of life with proper data migration and records retention. Strong requirements documentation also becomes the basis for later acceptance testing. Key concept: defining what the system must do, before design begins, is the requirements analysis phase of the SDLC.

Q11. A health system is selecting a new enterprise EHR and, after gathering its requirements, prepares a formal document inviting qualified vendors to describe in detail how their products satisfy the organization's functional and technical requirements, along with their proposed implementation approach, references, and pricing. The selection committee plans to score each vendor's response against weighted criteria so the decision is structured and defensible rather than based on impressions. This document is a:

A) Request for proposal (RFP)
B) Service level agreement (SLA)
C) Business associate agreement (BAA)
D) Memorandum of understanding (MOU)

Answer: A — A request for proposal (RFP) solicits detailed, structured vendor responses describing how each product meets stated requirements, typically including the proposed solution, implementation plan, references, and pricing, so responses can be scored and compared objectively against weighted selection criteria. It is more detailed than a request for information (RFI), which is used earlier to gather general market knowledge. A service level agreement (SLA) defines measurable performance and support commitments once a vendor is engaged. A business associate agreement (BAA) governs how a vendor handles PHI on the covered entity's behalf as required by HIPAA, and a memorandum of understanding (MOU) is a broad, often non-binding statement of mutual intent. Key concept: the RFP is the structured, scored solicitation used to compare competing vendor solutions during selection.

Q12. When a hospital migrates from an old patient-registration system to a new one, leadership decides to operate both systems at the same time for several weeks so that staff can verify the new system produces matching, correct results before the legacy system is retired. Which go-live (implementation) strategy is the hospital using?

A) Big bang
B) Parallel
C) Pilot
D) Rollback

Answer: B — A parallel implementation runs the legacy and new systems simultaneously so that outputs can be compared and validated before the old system is fully decommissioned, which lowers risk at the cost of duplicated effort and double the staff workload during the overlap period. A big-bang approach cuts over to the new system all at once on a single date, which is faster and cheaper but carries higher risk if problems surface. A pilot (or phased) approach deploys the new system to a limited unit or location first so lessons can be applied before broader rollout. Rollback is a contingency action to revert to the prior state if a deployment fails, not a planned go-live strategy; recognizing which approach trades risk for cost and effort is the key distinction here. Key concept: running old and new systems at the same time to verify results before retiring the old one is the parallel strategy.

Q13. Your team supports a middleware tool that sits in the middle of the hospital's systems and receives HL7 messages from the lab system, transforms certain fields into the formats each recipient expects, and routes copies to the EHR, the billing system, and a clinical data warehouse — all without each application having to connect directly to every other application. A colleague observes that without this tool, the number of point-to-point connections would balloon as systems were added. What is this integration component most commonly called?

A) Interface engine
B) Master patient index
C) Picture archiving and communication system (PACS)
D) Identity provider

Answer: A — An interface engine (also called an integration engine) receives messages such as HL7 V2, transforms and filters them, and routes them to multiple downstream systems, dramatically reducing the number of fragile point-to-point connections that would otherwise be required. Without it, connecting many systems directly to one another produces an unmanageable web of interfaces that grows quadratically; the hub-and-spoke model an interface engine provides simplifies maintenance, monitoring, and error handling. A master patient index reconciles patient identity across systems, a PACS stores and distributes medical images, and an identity provider authenticates users — none of which performs the message-routing function described here. Key concept: the interface (integration) engine is the middleware hub that transforms and routes messages among many systems.

Q14. A networking technician is walking you through the clinic's network closet as part of your orientation and points to a device whose job is to forward data packets between separate networks — for example, between the clinic's internal network and the internet — choosing the best path to each destination using its routing table.

The technician contrasts it with another box nearby that only moves traffic among devices inside the same local network. Which device is the technician describing as the one that connects and routes between networks?

A) Switch
B) Router
C) Hub
D) Firewall

Answer: B — A router operates primarily at the network layer (Layer 3) and forwards packets between different networks, selecting optimal paths using routing tables and routing protocols and connecting a local network to other networks such as the internet. A switch forwards frames intelligently among devices within the same local network using MAC addresses, while a hub is a legacy device that simply repeats incoming signals to all ports without any filtering or intelligence. A firewall enforces security policy by permitting or blocking traffic according to rules, but its primary role is protection, not inter-network path selection. Recognizing the router as the device that bridges and routes between networks is a foundational networking concept for health IT. Key concept: routers move packets between networks; switches move frames within a network.

Q15. While troubleshooting a connectivity issue on a nursing unit, a senior engineer explains that the workstation's logical network address keeps changing because it is assigned dynamically, so instead she asks you to identify the specific workstation by the unique hardware address that was permanently assigned to its network interface card at the time of manufacture. She says this address will reliably point to the same physical machine no matter what network it is plugged into. Which type of address are you being asked to find?

A) IP address
B) MAC address
C) URL
D) Port number

Answer: B — The Media Access Control (MAC) address is a unique hardware identifier assigned to a network interface card at the time of manufacture and used for communication within a local network segment at the data link layer (Layer 2). An IP address, by contrast, is a logical address that is configured statically or assigned dynamically via DHCP and can change depending on which network the device joins. A URL locates a web resource, and a port number identifies a particular application or service on a host. Distinguishing the permanent, manufacturer-assigned hardware address (MAC) from the changeable, network-assigned logical address (IP) is a common entry-level networking concept and useful when tracing a specific device on a network. Key concept: the MAC address is burned into the hardware; the IP address is assigned by the network.

Q16. A clinical data analyst is building a report that combines lab results from several hospitals and outside reference laboratories, but each source uses its own internal codes and names for the same tests, so the results will not line up. The analyst needs a standardized terminology to encode laboratory test orders and the resulting observations so that "serum glucose" from one lab and the equivalent test from another can be aggregated and compared reliably. Which standardized terminology is purpose-built for laboratory tests and clinical observations and measurements?

A) RxNorm
B) CPT
C) The SNOMED CT procedure hierarchy
D) LOINC

Answer: D — Logical Observation Identifiers Names and Codes (LOINC) is the standard terminology for identifying laboratory tests, clinical measurements, vital signs, and other observations, enabling consistent aggregation, comparison, and exchange of results across organizations regardless of the local names each lab uses. RxNorm standardizes clinical drug names, and CPT codes procedures and services for billing purposes. Although SNOMED CT is a broad clinical terminology that can represent many concepts, it is not the designated standard for naming laboratory observations and results — that is LOINC's specific role. USCDI references LOINC for laboratory data elements, which reinforces its position as the U.S. standard for observations. Key concept: when the question is about lab tests and the resulting observations, the standardized terminology is LOINC, which lets results from different labs be compared on common terms.

Q17. A pharmacy informatics team is building an interface between two systems that store medication names differently — one application records brand names while the other records generic ingredient names, so the same drug appears under two unrelated labels and automated reconciliation fails. They need a normalized naming system that links the various brand and generic representations of the same clinical drug so the systems can recognize them as equivalent. Which terminology should they use?

A) ICD-10-CM
B) RxNorm
C) LOINC
D) DICOM

Answer: B — RxNorm, produced by the National Library of Medicine, provides normalized names for clinical drugs and links many proprietary and source drug vocabularies, so systems that use different naming conventions for the same medication can interoperate reliably. This makes RxNorm central to e-prescribing, medication reconciliation, formulary management, and automated drug-interaction checking. ICD-10-CM codes diagnoses, LOINC codes laboratory and clinical observations, and DICOM is the standard for medical imaging objects and their communication. The exam frequently asks you to match each terminology to its domain: drugs to RxNorm, labs to LOINC, diagnoses to ICD, and broad clinical concepts to SNOMED CT. Key concept: RxNorm normalizes drug names and links brand and generic representations of the same medication.

Q18. A new associate keeps confusing several code systems — billing codes, messaging standards, and clinical terminologies — and asks you to clarify what SNOMED CT actually is and where it fits, because they have seen it referenced in documentation, decision-support rules, and analytics. You want to give them an accurate one-sentence characterization they can rely on. Which statement best characterizes SNOMED CT?

A) A billing code set used to submit professional service claims to payers
B) A comprehensive, hierarchically organized clinical terminology used to encode clinical findings, disorders, and procedures within the health record
C) A messaging standard for transmitting orders and results between systems
D) A federal regulation that governs breach notification timelines

Answer: B — SNOMED CT (Systematized Nomenclature of Medicine — Clinical Terms) is a comprehensive, multidisciplinary clinical terminology with a hierarchical, concept-oriented structure used to represent clinical content such as findings, disorders, body structures, organisms, and procedures within the electronic record. Because it is so granular and richly linked, it supports detailed clinical documentation, decision support, and analytics, and it can be mapped to billing code sets when needed. It is not itself a billing code set (CPT and ICD perform that role), not a messaging standard like HL7 or FHIR, and not a regulation. A useful mental model is that SNOMED CT captures *what the clinician means* clinically, while billing codes capture *what gets reimbursed*. Key concept: SNOMED CT is a comprehensive clinical terminology for documentation and decision support, not a billing or messaging standard.

Q19. A coding manager is training new staff and explains that in the United States, providers must use one specific standardized code set to report patient diagnoses — the reason a patient was seen or treated — both for clinical documentation and on the claims submitted to payers under the HIPAA transaction standards. She cautions the trainees not to confuse this diagnosis code set with the separate systems used for procedures, lab observations, or drug products. Which diagnosis code set is required for reporting diagnoses?

A) CPT
B) ICD-10-CM
C) LOINC
D) NDC

Answer: B — ICD-10-CM (International Classification of Diseases, 10th Revision, Clinical Modification) is the U.S. standard code set for reporting patient diagnoses in both clinical documentation and on claims under the HIPAA-adopted transaction standards, and it is maintained for U.S. use by the CDC's National Center for Health Statistics. CPT codes report procedures and professional services for billing, LOINC codes laboratory and clinical observations, and the National Drug Code (NDC) identifies specific drug products. Inpatient hospital procedures, separately, are coded with ICD-10-PCS rather than ICD-10-CM, so be careful not to confuse the diagnosis modification (CM) with the procedure coding system (PCS). Key concept: diagnoses on U.S. claims are reported with ICD-10-CM.

Q20. During a staff meeting, leadership references TEFCA — the Trusted Exchange Framework and Common Agreement — as a key federal effort to advance nationwide interoperability and to reduce the patchwork of one-off data-sharing agreements that organizations have historically negotiated separately. A colleague who is new to the topic asks you to summarize, in plain terms, what TEFCA actually does and how networks connect under it. Which statement best describes its purpose?

A) It defines a single new technical messaging standard that replaces FHIR for all exchange
B) It is the federal program that tests and certifies EHR software products

C) It establishes a common set of principles and a legal and technical framework that lets health information networks connect and exchange data, with Qualified Health Information Networks serving as the connective backbone
D) It is the HIPAA enforcement mechanism that assesses penalties for breaches

Answer: C — TEFCA creates a baseline of trust through common principles (the Trusted Exchange Framework) and a binding legal-and-technical agreement (the Common Agreement) that enable participating networks to interconnect, with Qualified Health Information Networks (QHINs) acting as the connective backbone that links exchange networks across the country. It is designed to reduce the patchwork of separate data-sharing agreements that organizations previously had to negotiate one by one. TEFCA complements existing standards such as FHIR rather than replacing them, and over time it incorporates FHIR-based exchange into its roadmap. It is distinct from ONC's Health IT Certification Program (which certifies software) and from HIPAA enforcement, which the HHS Office for Civil Rights handles. Key concept: TEFCA is a trust framework plus common agreement that connects networks through QHINs, not a new messaging standard.

Q21. A purchasing committee evaluating two EHR finalists wants independent assurance — not just the vendors' own marketing claims — that each candidate product has been verified to meet defined technical standards and interoperability capabilities such as standardized data export and API access. You point them to the ONC Health IT Certification Program as the appropriate source of that assurance. Which statement best describes the significance of that program?

A) It licenses individual clinicians to practice within a state
B) It tests and certifies that health IT products conform to adopted standards, implementation specifications, and certification criteria, including interoperability and API access requirements
C) It sets the reimbursement rates that hospitals receive for inpatient services
D) It accredits hospitals for Joint Commission status

Answer: B — The ONC Health IT Certification Program evaluates and certifies that health IT — most prominently EHR technology — conforms to adopted standards, implementation specifications, and certification criteria, including those supporting USCDI data, standardized FHIR-based API access, patient data export, and information-blocking-related capabilities. Testing is conducted by ONC-Authorized Testing and Certification Bodies, and choosing certified products gives organizations confidence in interoperability and regulatory alignment. The program does not license clinicians, set reimbursement rates, or perform hospital accreditation, which are functions of state licensing boards, CMS, and accrediting organizations such as The Joint Commission respectively. Certification is about the software's capabilities, not the providers who use it. Key concept: ONC certification verifies that health IT products meet adopted standards and criteria, including interoperability and API requirements.

Q22. A health system is rolling out a new EHR module that significantly changes how nurses document care, and leadership is worried that frontline staff will resist or work around the new screens if they are not brought along. The implementation plan therefore emphasizes engaging stakeholders early, clearly communicating the reasons for the change, providing thorough hands-on training, identifying unit "super users," and actively surfacing and addressing staff concerns and resistance throughout the transition. These activities are core to which discipline?

A) Penetration testing
B) Data warehousing
C) Capitation
D) Change management

Answer: D — Change management focuses on the people side of transitions — stakeholder engagement, transparent communication of the rationale, training, readiness assessment, and active management of resistance — so that new systems and workflows are actually adopted and sustained, not merely installed. Many health IT initiatives that are technically sound nonetheless fail on adoption, which is exactly why this discipline is emphasized in the CAHIMS leadership and administration domain. Penetration testing is a security assessment that probes for vulnerabilities, data warehousing is a data-architecture practice for analytics, and capitation is a fixed-per-member, per-period payment model. Of these, only change management addresses how people accept and use a new system. Key concept: stakeholder engagement, communication, and training to drive adoption are the heart of change management.

Q23. A covered entity discovers that an unencrypted laptop containing the protected health information of 700 patients has been stolen from an employee's parked car overnight. Because the device was not encrypted, the data is potentially readable by whoever has it, and the compliance team must now determine the organization's obligations under the HIPAA Breach Notification Rule, including whom to notify and how quickly. Which action is generally required?

A) No notification is required because fewer than 1,000 records were affected
B) Notify affected individuals without unreasonable delay and no later than 60 days from discovery, and notify the Secretary of HHS; because 500 or more individuals are affected, also provide prompt HHS and media notice
C) Notify only the laptop manufacturer and the device-management vendor
D) Wait to report the incident until the next scheduled annual compliance audit

Answer: B — The HIPAA Breach Notification Rule requires covered entities to notify affected individuals without unreasonable delay and no later than 60 days after discovery, and to notify the Secretary of HHS; breaches affecting 500 or more individuals additionally trigger notice to HHS without unreasonable delay (and no later than 60 days) and to prominent media outlets serving the affected area. Encryption that renders PHI unusable, unreadable, or indecipherable to unauthorized persons can qualify for a safe harbor and avoid notification — which is a strong reason to encrypt portable devices — but an unencrypted stolen laptop generally does not. There is no minimum record threshold that exempts smaller breaches from individual notification; the 500-person figure only changes the timing and breadth of regulator and media notice, not whether individuals must be told. Key concept: notify affected individuals and HHS within 60 days; encryption can provide a safe harbor that avoids notification altogether.

Q24. During a quarterly access review, your security lead notices that several registration clerks can open full clinical notes they never need, and insists that going forward each user account be configured to allow only the minimum information access necessary for that person to perform their specific job duties — and nothing more. The goal is to shrink the damage that any one compromised or misused account could do. Which security principle is being applied?

A) Least privilege
B) Defense in depth
C) Single sign-on
D) Data redundancy

Answer: A — The principle of least privilege limits every user's access rights to only what is required to perform their specific role, which reduces both the likelihood and the potential impact of accidental misuse, insider threat, or a compromised account being used to reach data it should never touch. It is a foundational access-control concept and pairs naturally with role-based access control and with HIPAA's "minimum necessary" standard. Defense in depth layers multiple independent controls so that no single failure exposes the system, single sign-on streamlines authentication across multiple systems for convenience, and data redundancy addresses availability and backup rather than access scope. Only least privilege directly answers the question of *how much* access each user should receive. Key concept: grant the minimum access necessary for the role — this is least privilege, closely aligned with HIPAA's minimum necessary standard.

Q25. After a series of phishing attempts in which stolen passwords were used to access clinical systems, an organization decides to strengthen log-in security for the EHR by requiring that users present a password plus a one-time code generated by a hardware token or a mobile authenticator app before they are granted access. The security team notes that even if an attacker steals the password, they still cannot log in without the second item. This control combines something the user knows with something the user has. What is this access control best described as?

A) Multi-factor authentication
B) Audit logging
C) Data encryption at rest
D) Network segmentation

Answer: A — Multi-factor authentication (MFA) requires two or more independent authentication factors drawn from different categories — typically combining something you know (a password), something you have (a hardware token or phone-based code), and something you are (a biometric) — which makes a stolen password far less useful to an attacker who lacks the second factor. Requiring a password plus a one-time code is a textbook example, because it pairs a knowledge factor with a possession factor. Audit logging records who did what and when, encryption at rest protects stored data from being read if media is lost, and network segmentation isolates portions of the network to contain threats. None of those three verifies a user's identity at log-in, which is the specific control the scenario describes. Key concept: combining factors from two different categories (know, have, are) is multi-factor authentication, and it is one of the most effective controls against stolen-password and phishing-based account takeovers.

Q26. A community hospital is moving its patient scheduling application to a vendor-hosted environment where the vendor manages the operating system, runtime, and the application itself, and the hospital simply logs in and configures workflows. Which cloud service model does this BEST describe?

A) Infrastructure as a Service (IaaS)
B) Platform as a Service (PaaS)
C) Software as a Service (SaaS)
D) On-premises hosting

Answer: C — In Software as a Service (SaaS), the vendor owns and manages the entire technology stack — physical infrastructure, networking, storage, operating system, runtime, and the application code — while the customer simply consumes the software through a browser or thin client and configures it to suit local workflows. Because the hospital only logs in and adjusts scheduling rules rather than patching servers or maintaining code, this scenario is the textbook definition of SaaS and is the most common cloud model for off-the-shelf clinical and administrative applications. With IaaS the hospital would receive raw virtual machines and remain responsible for the operating system and everything above it, and with PaaS it would receive a development and deployment platform on which its own staff build custom applications. On-premises hosting would place all hardware and software inside the hospital's own data center under its full control, which is the opposite of the vendor-managed arrangement described here.

Q27. A CAHIMS-credentialed analyst is asked to explain the practical benefit of telehealth for a rural critical access hospital that has difficulty recruiting specialists. Which statement describes the MOST appropriate benefit to communicate?

A) Telehealth eliminates the need for any in-person clinical encounters
B) Telehealth removes all licensure and credentialing requirements for remote providers
C) Telehealth extends specialty access to patients who would otherwise travel long distances to see a specialist
D) Telehealth guarantees lower costs in every clinical scenario

Answer: C — The defining value of telehealth in a rural or underserved setting is its ability to extend access to specialty expertise that is not locally available, sparing patients long and sometimes prohibitive travel and reducing dangerous delays in diagnosis and treatment. Telehealth supplements in-person care rather than replacing it, since many conditions still require hands-on examination, imaging, or procedures, so claiming it eliminates physical encounters would be inaccurate and would set unrealistic expectations. Remote providers also remain subject to licensure in the patient's state and to facility credentialing requirements, frequently satisfied through credentialing-by-proxy arrangements between the originating and distant sites. Cost outcomes vary widely by use case, reimbursement model, and technology investment, so promising universal savings would overstate the benefit and could mislead leadership during planning.

Q28. An organization is implementing a machine learning model that predicts which patients are at high risk for hospital readmission. During validation, the team notices the model performs noticeably worse for one demographic subgroup than for others. According to responsible AI practice, what is the MOST appropriate next step?

A) Deploy the model anyway because overall accuracy is acceptable
B) Investigate the model for bias and evaluate the representativeness of the training data before deployment
C) Remove the underperforming subgroup from the patient population
D) Increase the model's confidence threshold for all patients equally

Answer: B — A measurable performance gap across demographic subgroups is one of the clearest warning signs of algorithmic bias, which frequently originates in training data that under-represents, mislabels, or systematically skews certain populations. Responsible AI practice requires investigating the root cause of the disparity and assessing whether the training data adequately represents the patients the model will serve before the model is allowed to influence care decisions. Deploying despite the gap would risk propagating inequitable care to a vulnerable group, removing the affected subgroup from the analysis simply hides the patients who most need accurate predictions, and uniformly raising the confidence threshold does nothing to correct an underlying representational bias. Surfacing and remediating bias before go-live protects both patients and the organization's clinical, legal, and ethical obligations.

Q29. During a security awareness training session, an employee asks which element of the CIA triad is primarily protected when an organization uses access controls and encryption to prevent unauthorized people from viewing patient records. Which element is BEST described?

A) Confidentiality
B) Integrity
C) Availability
D) Accountability

Answer: A — Confidentiality is the security principle of ensuring that information is disclosed only to individuals, entities, or processes authorized to access it, and access controls together with encryption are the canonical safeguards that enforce it. By restricting who can view patient records and rendering any intercepted data unreadable without the proper key, the organization is directly protecting confidentiality. Integrity, the second element of the triad, concerns the accuracy and trustworthiness of data and its protection from unauthorized alteration or destruction, while availability, the third element, ensures that systems and data are accessible to authorized users when needed. Accountability, although a vital security concept that ties actions to identities, is not one of the three components of the CIA triad and is therefore the wrong choice here.

Q30. A health system is rolling out multi-factor authentication (MFA) for remote access to its electronic health record. A clinician asks why a password alone is no longer sufficient. Which explanation is MOST accurate?

A) MFA replaces the password with a single biometric so the user no longer needs to remember anything
B) MFA requires two or more independent factors, such as something you know and something you have, making stolen passwords far less useful to an attacker
C) MFA encrypts the password so it cannot be intercepted
D) MFA is required only for administrators, not clinical staff

Answer: B — Multi-factor authentication combines two or more independent categories of credentials — typically something you know (a password or PIN), something you have (a hardware token, smartphone, or one-time code), and something you are (a fingerprint or facial scan). The strength of MFA comes from this independence: even if an attacker phishes, guesses, or buys a password, they still lack the second factor and cannot complete the login, which sharply reduces account compromise. MFA supplements rather than replaces the password, so it does not eliminate the need to remember credentials, and it does not by itself encrypt the password as it travels across the network. Because remote access to an EHR exposes large volumes of protected health information, MFA is broadly recommended and increasingly required for all users with such access, not only administrators.

Q31. A staff member receives an email that appears to come from the IT help desk, urgently asking them to click a link and re-enter their network credentials to avoid account suspension. The email address contains subtle misspellings. This is an example of which type of threat?

A) Ransomware
B) Phishing
C) Denial-of-service attack
D) SQL injection

Answer: B — Phishing is a social engineering attack in which an adversary impersonates a trusted entity — such as an internal help desk — to manipulate users into revealing credentials, clicking malicious links, or disclosing sensitive information. The hallmarks present here are unmistakable: a sense of manufactured urgency ("avoid account suspension"), a request to re-enter credentials, and a sender address with subtle misspellings designed to mimic a legitimate domain. Ransomware encrypts an organization's data and demands payment for its release, a denial-of-service attack floods systems with traffic to make them unavailable, and SQL injection inserts malicious code into a database query. None of those alternatives describe a credential-harvesting lure delivered by email, which makes phishing the correct classification and a key topic in every security awareness program.

Q32. A hospital's security team is configuring user accounts so that each employee can access only the systems and data necessary to perform their specific job duties. Which security principle are they applying?

A) Defense in depth
B) Least privilege
C) Separation of duties
D) Non-repudiation

Answer: B — The principle of least privilege holds that users, processes, and systems should be granted only the minimum access rights required to perform their legitimate functions and nothing more, which limits the potential damage from compromised, stolen, or misused accounts. By scoping each employee's access strictly to what their role requires — often implemented through role-based access control — the security team is applying least privilege directly. Defense in depth refers to layering multiple, overlapping controls so that the failure of one does not expose the whole system, and separation of duties divides a single critical task among multiple individuals to prevent fraud or error by any one person. Non-repudiation ensures that an actor cannot credibly deny having performed a recorded action and is unrelated to the provisioning of minimal access.

Q33. A ransomware attack has encrypted several departmental file servers, and clinical staff cannot access electronic documents. Which preparedness measure would have BEST enabled the organization to recover its data without paying the ransom?

A) A stronger firewall configured after the attack
B) Tested, offline backups of critical data maintained on a regular schedule
C) A longer password policy implemented going forward
D) Disabling all email accounts during the incident

Answer: B — Maintaining regular backups that are tested for restorability and stored offline or otherwise isolated from the production network is the single most effective defense for ransomware recovery, because it allows the organization to wipe affected systems and restore clean data rather than negotiate with attackers. The "tested" qualifier is essential: many organizations discover during a crisis that their backups are corrupt, incomplete, or themselves encrypted because they were left continuously connected to the network. A firewall configured after the fact and a stronger password policy may help prevent the next attack but cannot recover data that is already encrypted, and disabling email mid-incident neither restores files nor addresses the encryption. Resilient, isolated, verified backups are the recovery control that breaks the attacker's extortion leverage.

Q34. A nurse manager wants a single screen that displays real-time bed occupancy, average wait times, and staffing ratios so she can make quick operational decisions during a busy shift. Which analytics tool BEST meets this need?

A) A static annual report
B) An operational dashboard with key performance indicators
C) A raw data export to a spreadsheet
D) A predictive model trained on historical admissions

Answer: B — An operational dashboard consolidates real-time or near-real-time key performance indicators into a single visual display, allowing managers to monitor current conditions at a glance and act quickly on emerging issues such as bed shortages or staffing imbalances. Its strength is timeliness and visual consolidation precisely matched to the in-the-moment decisions a nurse manager makes during a busy shift. A static annual report reflects a fixed point in the past and cannot guide live operations, while a raw spreadsheet export forces the manager to do her own analysis and lacks the at-a-glance usability she needs. A predictive model forecasts likely future states rather than displaying the current operational picture, so the operational dashboard is the tool purpose-built for this real-time monitoring scenario.

Q35. An analytics team is asked to distinguish between descriptive and predictive analytics for a leadership briefing. Which pairing correctly matches each type to its purpose?

A) Descriptive forecasts future events; predictive summarizes what already happened
B) Descriptive summarizes what has already happened; predictive estimates what is likely to happen
C) Both describe only historical data
D) Both forecast future outcomes using machine learning

Answer: B — Descriptive analytics summarizes and reports on historical and current data — answering the question "what happened" — through metrics, aggregations, reports, and visualizations that establish a factual baseline. Predictive analytics builds on that foundation by applying statistical methods and machine learning to historical patterns in order to estimate the probability of future outcomes, answering "what is likely to happen." These two sit at different points on the analytics maturity continuum, with prescriptive analytics ("what should we do about it") extending beyond them. Reversing the definitions, claiming both are limited to history, or claiming both forecast the future each misrepresents the distinct and complementary roles these analytic types play in supporting data-driven decisions.

Q36. A project manager is building a RACI chart for an EHR optimization project. A stakeholder asks what the "A" designation means for a given task. Which definition is correct?

A) The person who performs the work
B) The single person ultimately answerable for the task's completion and correctness
C) Anyone whose input is sought before a decision
D) Anyone who is kept informed of progress

Answer: B — In a RACI responsibility matrix, the "A" stands for Accountable, designating the one individual who is ultimately answerable for a task being completed correctly and on time, and who holds the authority to approve the work. A core rule of RACI is that each task has exactly one Accountable party, because splitting accountability creates ambiguity about who truly owns the outcome. The "R" (Responsible) identifies the people who actually perform the work, the "C" (Consulted) identifies those whose subject-matter input is sought through two-way dialogue before decisions, and the "I" (Informed) identifies those who are kept updated through one-way communication. Clearly assigning the single Accountable owner is the chart's central organizing purpose and a frequent source of confusion that the tool is designed to resolve.

Q37. A team is decomposing a large EHR implementation into smaller, manageable deliverables and sub-deliverables organized hierarchically to clarify scope and assign work. Which project management tool are they creating?

A) A Gantt chart
B) A work breakdown structure (WBS)
C) A risk register
D) A stakeholder matrix

Answer: B — A work breakdown structure (WBS) is a hierarchical, deliverable-oriented decomposition of the total project scope into progressively smaller components and work packages, giving the team a clear and complete picture of everything that must be produced. By breaking a large EHR implementation into discrete deliverables and sub-deliverables, the team can estimate effort, sequence work, and assign responsibility with far greater precision. A Gantt chart visualizes the project schedule and task dependencies across a timeline rather than decomposing scope, a risk register catalogs identified risks along with their likelihood, impact, and response plans, and a stakeholder matrix maps interested parties and their influence. Only the WBS specifically organizes the work itself into a manageable hierarchy of deliverables, which is exactly what the team is building.

Q38. A hospital IT department is choosing between Agile and waterfall methodologies for a project where requirements are expected to evolve and frequent stakeholder feedback is desired. Which methodology is generally BEST suited, and why?

A) Waterfall, because it allows requirements to change at any phase
B) Agile, because it delivers work in iterative increments and accommodates changing requirements through frequent feedback
C) Waterfall, because it relies on continuous stakeholder collaboration each sprint
D) Agile, because it requires all requirements to be fully fixed before development begins

Answer: B — Agile methodologies deliver work in short, iterative increments called sprints and explicitly embrace changing requirements, using frequent demonstrations and stakeholder feedback to adjust direction as understanding deepens over the life of the project. This makes Agile well suited to initiatives whose requirements are expected to evolve and where ongoing collaboration is valued, exactly as described here. Waterfall, by contrast, proceeds sequentially through fixed phases — requirements, design, build, test, deploy — and works best when requirements are well understood and stable up front, because changes introduced late in a waterfall project are expensive and disruptive. The distractor options misattribute Agile's flexibility and sprint-based collaboration to waterfall and falsely claim Agile demands fully fixed requirements, so the correctly reasoned choice is Agile delivered in iterative increments.

Q39. During interoperability planning, an analyst needs to recommend a modern, web-based standard that uses RESTful APIs and structured resources to exchange discrete healthcare data between systems. Which standard should the analyst recommend?

A) HL7 FHIR (Fast Healthcare Interoperability Resources)
B) DICOM
C) NCPDP SCRIPT
D) X12 EDI

Answer: A — HL7 FHIR (Fast Healthcare Interoperability Resources) is the contemporary interoperability standard built on familiar web technologies, exposing healthcare data as modular "resources" — such as Patient, Observation, and Medication — that can be exchanged through RESTful APIs. Its API-driven, resource-based design supports flexible, app-based access to discrete data elements, which is exactly what modern interoperability initiatives and the federal information-sharing requirements of the 21st Century Cures Act call for. DICOM is the standard governing the storage and transmission of medical images, NCPDP SCRIPT handles electronic prescribing transactions between prescribers and pharmacies, and X12 EDI governs administrative transactions such as claims, eligibility, and remittance advice. For exchanging structured clinical data through web APIs, FHIR is the clear and current recommendation.

Q40. A regional collection of hospitals and clinics wants to share patient data electronically so that a treating clinician can retrieve records from any participating organization. Which entity facilitates this exchange?
A) A health information exchange (HIE)
B) A picture archiving and communication system (PACS)
C) A clearinghouse for claims
D) A computerized provider order entry (CPOE) system

Answer: A — A health information exchange (HIE) is an organization or network that enables the secure electronic sharing of patient health information among participating providers and organizations across a region or community, supporting continuity of care when a patient is seen in multiple settings. Through an HIE, a treating clinician can retrieve records that originated at other participating facilities, which improves care coordination and reduces duplicate testing and conflicting treatment. A picture archiving and communication system stores and retrieves medical images within an organization, a claims clearinghouse routes and standardizes billing transactions between providers and payers, and a CPOE system lets providers enter clinical orders electronically. Only the HIE performs the cross-organizational clinical data-sharing function described in the scenario.

Q41. A CAHIMS candidate is studying the framework established to create a nationwide floor for interoperability that connects health information networks through common rules and a single on-ramp. Which initiative does this describe?
A) Meaningful Use Stage 1
B) The Trusted Exchange Framework and Common Agreement (TEFCA)
C) The HIPAA Privacy Rule
D) ICD-10-CM coding

Answer: B — The Trusted Exchange Framework and Common Agreement (TEFCA) establishes a common set of principles, terms, and conditions that allow health information networks to connect to one another nationwide through participating Qualified Health Information Networks, creating a universal floor for interoperability and a simplified on-ramp for data exchange. Its purpose is to enable trusted, secure exchange across previously siloed networks under shared governance and consistent rules. Meaningful Use Stage 1 was an early phase of the EHR incentive program promoting basic certified-EHR adoption, the HIPAA Privacy Rule governs how protected health information may be used and disclosed, and ICD-10-CM is a clinical diagnosis coding system. Only TEFCA defines the nationwide trusted-exchange infrastructure that the question describes.

Q42. A data governance committee discovers that a patient's date of birth is recorded differently in three systems. They want a single dimension of data quality to label this problem. Which dimension is MOST directly affected?
A) Timeliness
B) Consistency
C) Completeness
D) Granularity

Answer: B — Consistency is the data quality dimension concerned with whether a given data element holds the same value across different systems, records, and points in time; three systems showing different dates of birth for the same patient is a classic consistency failure. Inconsistent values undermine trust in the data and can cause clinical errors and identity-matching problems, which is why governance committees prioritize reconciling them. Timeliness addresses whether data is sufficiently current for its intended use, completeness addresses whether all required data elements are present, and granularity addresses whether data is captured at an appropriate level of detail. Because the issue here is conflicting values for the same field rather than missing, stale, or under-detailed data, consistency is the most directly affected dimension.

Q43. A quality analyst finds that 8 percent of patient records are missing a documented primary language. Which data quality dimension does this gap MOST directly represent?
A) Accuracy
B) Completeness
C) Validity
D) Uniqueness

Answer: B — Completeness measures whether all required or expected data elements are present within a record or dataset; missing primary-language entries in 8 percent of records is a straightforward completeness deficiency. Completeness gaps matter operationally because absent fields can prevent appropriate interpreter services, accurate population-health analytics, and required regulatory reporting. Accuracy concerns whether recorded values are factually correct, validity concerns whether values conform to defined formats or permitted value ranges, and uniqueness concerns the absence of duplicate records for the same entity. Because the problem described is the absence of data rather than wrong, malformed, or duplicated data, completeness is the precise dimension at issue and the one the analyst should cite.

Q44. A hospital's EHR will be unavailable for four hours during a planned upgrade. Which measure BEST ensures that clinical care can continue safely during this period?

A) Postponing all patient care until the system returns
B) Activating established downtime procedures, including paper forms and read-only access to recent data
C) Granting all staff administrator rights during the outage
D) Disabling the backup systems to speed the upgrade

Answer: B — Established downtime procedures — including standardized paper documentation forms, predefined clinical workflows, and business continuity access that provides read-only copies of recent patient data — allow clinicians to continue delivering safe care while the EHR is unavailable, whether the outage is planned or unplanned. These procedures should be documented, regularly rehearsed, and supported by clear staff roles so the transition into and out of downtime is orderly and reconciliation afterward is reliable. Postponing all care is unsafe and frequently impossible in a hospital setting, granting blanket administrator rights introduces serious security and data-integrity risks, and disabling backups removes a critical safety net at the worst possible moment. Well-prepared downtime procedures are the standard preparedness control for maintaining continuity of care during system outages.

Q45. Under the HIPAA Breach Notification Rule, when a breach of unsecured protected health information affects 500 or more individuals in a single jurisdiction, which notification requirement applies?

A) Only the affected individuals must be notified, with no government reporting
B) Affected individuals, the Secretary of HHS, and prominent media outlets serving the area must be notified without unreasonable delay
C) Notification can be delayed up to one year
D) Notification is required only if financial harm is proven

Answer: B — When a breach of unsecured protected health information affects 500 or more residents of a state or jurisdiction, the HIPAA Breach Notification Rule requires the covered entity to notify the affected individuals, to notify the Secretary of Health and Human Services contemporaneously, and to notify prominent media outlets serving the affected area, all without unreasonable delay and no later than 60 days from discovery. Breaches affecting fewer than 500 individuals are instead reported to HHS on an annual basis, which is why the 500-individual threshold is a critical exam concept to memorize. An impermissible use or disclosure of unsecured PHI is presumed to be a reportable breach unless a documented risk assessment demonstrates a low probability that the information was compromised, so proof of financial harm is not a precondition for notification. The one-year delay option does not exist under the rule, making the media-and-HHS notification requirement the correct answer.

Q46. A covered entity must notify affected individuals of a breach of unsecured PHI within a defined outer time limit from the date of discovery. What is that maximum time frame under the HIPAA Breach Notification Rule?

A) 30 days
B) 60 days
C) 90 days
D) 180 days

Answer: B — The HIPAA Breach Notification Rule requires covered entities to notify affected individuals without unreasonable delay and in no case later than 60 calendar days following discovery of the breach. The discovery clock begins on the first day the breach is known, or reasonably should have been known, to the covered entity or any member of its workforce other than the person who committed the breach. The phrase "without unreasonable delay" is significant: organizations are expected to notify as soon as practicable and may not simply wait out the full 60 days when they are able to act sooner. The other intervals listed do not correspond to the regulatory standard, making 60 days the correct outer limit for individual notification.

Q47. A business associate experiences a breach of unsecured PHI that it maintains on behalf of a covered entity. What is the business associate's primary obligation under HIPAA?

A) Notify the affected patients directly and assume full responsibility
B) Notify the covered entity of the breach so the covered entity can fulfill its notification obligations
C) Take no action because only covered entities must report breaches
D) Notify only the media

Answer: B — Under HIPAA, a business associate that discovers a breach of unsecured PHI must notify the covered entity, generally without unreasonable delay and no later than 60 days from discovery, supplying the details — such as the individuals affected and the nature of the incident — that the covered entity needs to carry out its own notification duties. The covered entity, not the business associate, is ordinarily responsible for notifying affected individuals, HHS, and the media, unless the business associate agreement specifically delegates those tasks to the business associate. Taking no action would violate both the Breach Notification Rule and the business associate agreement, and a business associate that notified only the media while bypassing the covered entity would leave the actual regulatory obligations unmet. Prompt notification up the chain to the covered entity is therefore the business associate's core breach-response duty.

Q48. A health system is evaluating a hybrid cloud strategy that keeps sensitive PHI workloads on a private, internally controlled environment while using a public cloud for elastic, non-sensitive analytics workloads. What is the PRIMARY advantage of this hybrid approach?

A) It eliminates the need for any security controls
B) It balances control over sensitive data with the scalability and cost flexibility of public cloud resources
C) It guarantees the organization never has to manage any infrastructure
D) It removes all regulatory obligations for data stored in the public cloud

Answer: B — A hybrid cloud combines private and public cloud resources so an organization can place sensitive or tightly regulated workloads in a controlled private environment while taking advantage of the elasticity, on-demand scaling, and cost efficiency of public cloud for less sensitive workloads. This deliberate balance between control and flexibility is the primary advantage and the reason many health systems adopt hybrid architectures rather than going all-private or all-public. Hybrid cloud does not eliminate the need for security controls — in fact it requires consistent safeguards spanning both environments and the connections between them — and it does not free the organization from managing infrastructure, since the private portion still demands active stewardship. Most importantly, HIPAA and other regulatory obligations follow the PHI wherever it resides, so storing data in the public cloud never removes those duties, and appropriate business associate agreements and safeguards remain mandatory.

Q49. A hospital is deploying an AI-based clinical decision support tool and wants to ensure ongoing oversight after go-live. Which practice BEST supports responsible, sustained use of the model?

A) Validate the model once before deployment and assume performance remains stable indefinitely
B) Continuously monitor model performance for drift and bias and retrain or recalibrate as needed
C) Allow the model to make autonomous treatment decisions without clinician review
D) Hide the model's recommendations from clinicians to avoid bias

Answer: B — Responsible AI governance requires continuous post-deployment monitoring because a model's performance can degrade over time as patient populations, clinical practices, documentation patterns, and underlying data distributions shift — a phenomenon known as model drift — and because bias can emerge or intensify after go-live. Monitoring for drift and bias, paired with retraining or recalibration when performance falls outside acceptable bounds, sustains the tool's safety, accuracy, and fairness across its operational life. A one-time validation ignores drift and provides false assurance, allowing the model to make autonomous treatment decisions removes the essential human oversight that decision support is meant to augment rather than replace, and hiding the recommendations defeats the tool's purpose without doing anything to address bias. Ongoing surveillance combined with clinician review is the sound governance practice for sustained, responsible use.

Q50. A new CAHIMS-credentialed professional is asked to describe the value of strong governance and leadership engagement in a health IT project. Which statement BEST reflects an effective leadership and administration principle?

A) IT projects succeed primarily through technology selection, with minimal need for stakeholder communication
B) Clear governance, executive sponsorship, and stakeholder engagement are critical to aligning the project with organizational goals and securing adoption
C) Change management is unnecessary once the system is technically installed
D) Decisions should be made solely by the IT department without clinical input

Answer: B — Effective health IT initiatives depend on strong governance structures, visible executive sponsorship, and active stakeholder engagement to align the project with strategic objectives, allocate resources, resolve cross-departmental conflicts, and drive user adoption. Leadership engagement signals organizational commitment and provides the authority needed to remove barriers and sustain momentum when challenges arise. Technology selection alone does not ensure success, because even excellent systems fail when users are unprepared or unwilling to adopt them, and change management remains essential well past the technical installation to support workflow redesign, training, and reinforcement. Excluding clinical input would undermine usability, safety, and acceptance, so collaborative governance that engages clinical and operational stakeholders is the sound leadership and administration principle that a CAHIMS professional should articulate.

.46 Glossary of Key Terms

Agile. A project management and software development approach that delivers work in short, iterative cycles with continuous stakeholder feedback rather than a single linear sequence. In healthcare IT, Agile methods are increasingly used for configuration, dashboard, and interface projects where requirements evolve. Contrast with the traditional waterfall model embodied in the SDLC.

AI/ML (Artificial Intelligence / Machine Learning). AI refers to computer systems that perform tasks normally requiring human intelligence; machine learning is the subset in which algorithms learn patterns from data without explicit programming. In healthcare, AI/ML powers clinical decision support, risk prediction, image analysis, and ambient documentation. CAHIMS candidates should understand that AI tools raise governance, bias, validation, and regulatory questions, and that some qualify as Software as a Medical Device.

Big-Bang Implementation. A go-live strategy in which all modules, departments, or facilities transition to the new system simultaneously on a single cutover date. It is faster and avoids prolonged dual-system operation but concentrates risk and requires extensive command-center support. Contrast with the phased rollout approach.

Breach. Under HIPAA, the acquisition, access, use, or disclosure of protected health information in a manner not permitted by the Privacy Rule that compromises its security or privacy. Covered entities must conduct a risk assessment and, unless a low probability of compromise is demonstrated, notify affected individuals, the Department of Health and Human Services, and sometimes the media under the Breach Notification Rule.

CDA (Clinical Document Architecture). An HL7 XML-based markup standard that specifies the structure and semantics of clinical documents such as discharge summaries and progress notes for exchange. The Consolidated CDA (C-CDA) is the constrained implementation widely required for certified EHR document exchange. CDA documents are human-readable and machine-processable.

CDS (Clinical Decision Support). Technology that provides clinicians, staff, or patients with knowledge and person-specific information, intelligently filtered and presented at appropriate times, to enhance care. Common forms include drug-interaction alerts, order sets, reminders, and best-practice advisories. Poorly tuned CDS causes alert fatigue, a key usability and safety concern.

Charter (Project Charter). A formal document that authorizes a project, names the project manager, and defines high-level objectives, scope, stakeholders, milestones, and success criteria. It is typically produced during project initiation and grants authority to apply organizational resources. The charter aligns sponsors and the team before detailed planning begins.

CIA Triad. The foundational information-security model comprising Confidentiality (preventing unauthorized disclosure), Integrity (preventing unauthorized or improper alteration), and Availability (ensuring authorized access when needed). Every security control in a healthcare environment supports one or more of these goals. The triad frames HIPAA Security Rule safeguards.

Cloud (IaaS/PaaS/SaaS). Cloud computing delivers IT resources over the internet on demand. Infrastructure as a Service (IaaS) provides virtualized servers, storage, and networking; Platform as a Service (PaaS) adds development and deployment environments; Software as a Service (SaaS) delivers ready-to-use applications such as a hosted EHR. Each model shifts a different share of responsibility from the customer to the provider, with security obligations divided under a shared-responsibility framework.

CMS (Centers for Medicare & Medicaid Services). The federal agency within Health and Human Services that administers Medicare, Medicaid, and the Children's Health Insurance Program and sets many reimbursement and quality-reporting rules. CMS programs such as the Promoting Interoperability and Merit-based Incentive Payment System drive much EHR adoption and data reporting. CMS regulations frequently shape healthcare IT priorities.

CPOE (Computerized Provider Order Entry). The electronic entry of medication, laboratory, imaging, and other orders directly by the ordering clinician, replacing handwritten or verbal orders. CPOE reduces transcription errors and enables real-time clinical decision support and order sets. It is a core certified-EHR function and a patient-safety cornerstone.

Critical Path. In project scheduling, the longest sequence of dependent activities that determines the minimum project duration; any delay on a critical-path task delays the whole project. Identifying it lets the project manager focus monitoring and resources where slippage matters most. Tasks not on the critical path have float, or schedule slack.

Dashboard. A visual display that consolidates and presents key metrics and indicators on a single screen for at-a-glance monitoring. In healthcare IT, dashboards surface operational, clinical, and financial KPIs to support timely decisions. Effective dashboards are role-specific, current, and actionable rather than merely decorative.

Data Dictionary. A centralized repository of metadata that defines each data element in a system, including its name, type, allowable values, format, and meaning. It promotes consistency, supports interoperability, and is essential for analytics and integration projects. A shared data dictionary prevents the same field from being interpreted differently across teams.

Data Governance. The framework of policies, roles, standards, and processes that ensures data is accurate, secure, available, and used appropriately across an organization. It assigns accountability for data quality and stewardship and underpins trustworthy analytics and reporting. Strong governance is a prerequisite for reliable population-health and quality measurement.

Data Warehouse. A centralized repository that aggregates and stores integrated, historical data from multiple source systems, optimized for query, reporting, and analytics rather than transaction processing. Data is typically loaded through ETL processes and structured for efficient analysis. Warehouses enable enterprise reporting that operational EHR databases cannot easily support.

Downtime Procedure. Documented contingency plans and manual workflows that allow clinical and business operations to continue when an information system is unavailable, whether planned or unplanned. Components include paper forms, read-only backup access, and recovery steps to reconcile data once systems return. The HIPAA Security Rule requires a contingency plan including data backup, disaster recovery, and emergency-mode operation.

eMAR (Electronic Medication Administration Record). An electronic record documenting the administration of medications to patients, often integrated with barcode scanning of the patient and drug to verify the "rights" of medication administration. The eMAR closes the medication-management loop initiated by CPOE and pharmacy verification. It reduces administration errors and provides a real-time medication audit trail.

Encryption. The process of converting readable data into ciphertext using an algorithm and key so that only authorized parties with the key can decrypt it. The HIPAA Security Rule designates encryption an addressable implementation specification, and properly encrypted PHI may qualify for breach-notification safe harbor. Both data at rest and data in transit should be encrypted.

ePHI (Electronic Protected Health Information). Protected health information that is created, received, stored, or transmitted in electronic form. ePHI is the specific focus of the HIPAA Security Rule, which mandates administrative, physical, and technical safeguards. All identifiable electronic patient data within EHRs, portals, and devices is ePHI.

ETL (Extract, Transform, Load). The data-integration process of extracting data from source systems, transforming it into a consistent format and applying business rules, and loading it into a target such as a data warehouse. ETL ensures that aggregated analytics data is clean, standardized, and reliable. A related variant, ELT, loads data before transforming it within the target platform.

FHIR (Fast Healthcare Interoperability Resources). A modern HL7 interoperability standard that represents clinical and administrative data as modular "resources" exchanged over web-based RESTful APIs. FHIR underlies modern app ecosystems, including SMART on FHIR, and is required by ONC certification for standardized API access. Its API approach makes data exchange faster and more developer-friendly than older messaging standards.

Go-Live. The point at which a new or upgraded information system becomes operational and is used for actual patient care or business activity. Go-live is supported by training, command centers, at-the-elbow support, and downtime contingencies. Success depends on thorough planning, testing, and change management completed beforehand.

HIE (Health Information Exchange). Both the act of electronically sharing health information across organizations and the organizational entity (an HIE) that facilitates such sharing within a region or community. HIEs improve care coordination, reduce duplicate testing, and support public-health reporting. They are increasingly connected through national frameworks such as TEFCA.

HIPAA Privacy Rule. The federal regulation establishing national standards for protecting individuals' identifiable health information and governing its use and disclosure by covered entities and business associates. It grants patients rights to access, amend, and obtain an accounting of disclosures of their records and limits uses to the "minimum necessary." It applies to PHI in any form—oral, paper, or electronic.

HIPAA Security Rule. The federal regulation requiring covered entities and business associates to protect electronic protected health information through administrative, physical, and technical safeguards. It mandates a risk analysis and reasonable, appropriate controls, distinguishing "required" from "addressable" implementation specifications. The Security Rule operationalizes the CIA triad for ePHI.

HL7 v2 (Health Level Seven Version 2). A long-established messaging standard using pipe-and-hat delimited segments to exchange clinical and administrative data, such as admission, discharge, transfer, lab, and order messages, between systems. Despite its age and implementation variability, HL7 v2 remains the most widely deployed interface standard in hospitals. It coexists with newer standards like FHIR during ongoing modernization.

ICD-10-CM (International Classification of Diseases, 10th Revision, Clinical Modification). The U.S. code set for reporting diagnoses and conditions in healthcare settings, maintained for clinical and billing use. Its granular, alphanumeric codes support reimbursement, epidemiology, and quality measurement. ICD-10-CM is distinct from the procedure code set ICD-10-PCS used for inpatient procedures.

Information Blocking. Under the 21st Century Cures Act and ONC rules, a practice by a provider, health IT developer, or HIE that is likely to interfere with the access, exchange, or use of electronic health information, except as required by law or covered by a defined exception. Engaging in information blocking can trigger penalties and disincentives. The rule promotes patient and provider access to electronic health information.

Interoperability. The ability of different information systems, devices, and applications to access, exchange, integrate, and cooperatively use data in a coordinated manner across organizational and vendor boundaries. It is commonly described in foundational, structural, and semantic levels, with semantic interoperability requiring shared meaning through standardized terminologies. Achieving it is a central goal of healthcare IT standards and policy.

KPI (Key Performance Indicator). A quantifiable measure used to evaluate progress toward a specific objective or the performance of a process, department, or organization. In healthcare IT, KPIs include metrics such as portal adoption, system uptime, order-entry rates, and average length of stay. Good KPIs are specific, measurable, and tied to strategic goals.

Least Privilege. A security principle granting each user, process, or system only the minimum access rights necessary to perform their function, and no more. Applied through role-based access controls, it limits the damage from compromised accounts or insider misuse. It directly supports the HIPAA "minimum necessary" standard for ePHI.

LOINC (Logical Observation Identifiers Names and Codes). A universal terminology standard for identifying laboratory tests, clinical observations, and measurements, enabling consistent exchange of results across systems. Each LOINC code uniquely names what was measured, independent of the local lab's naming conventions. It is a named standard within USCDI and is essential for semantic interoperability of results.

Medication Reconciliation. The process of creating and maintaining the most accurate possible list of all medications a patient is taking and comparing it against orders at transitions of care such as admission, transfer, and discharge. It aims to prevent omissions, duplications, dosing errors, and harmful interactions. EHR tools support reconciliation but require disciplined clinical workflow to be effective.

MFA (Multi-Factor Authentication). An access-control method requiring two or more independent credentials from different categories—something you know, something you have, and something you are—before granting system access. MFA substantially reduces the risk of compromised passwords leading to unauthorized PHI access. It is a widely recommended technical safeguard for healthcare systems.

ONC Certification. The Office of the National Coordinator for Health Information Technology administers a program certifying that health IT meets standardized criteria for functionality, interoperability, and security. Certified EHR technology is required for participation in many CMS incentive and reporting programs. Certification criteria evolve, incorporating standards such as FHIR APIs and USCDI.

Patient Portal. A secure online application that gives patients access to portions of their health record, including results, visit summaries, medications, secure messaging, appointment scheduling, and bill payment. Portals support patient engagement and satisfy access requirements under the Cures Act and ONC rules. Portal adoption rates are a common engagement KPI.

Phased Implementation. A go-live strategy that introduces a new system incrementally—by module, department, or location—over time rather than all at once. It reduces risk and allows lessons to be applied to later phases but lengthens the timeline and may require temporary interfaces between old and new systems. Contrast with the big-bang approach.

PHI (Protected Health Information). Individually identifiable health information held or transmitted by a covered entity or business associate in any form—electronic, paper, or oral—that relates to a person's health, care, or payment. HIPAA identifies eighteen identifiers, such as name, dates, and medical record numbers, that render data PHI. Removing all identifiers (de-identification) takes data outside HIPAA's scope.

Problem List. A current, structured summary of a patient's significant diagnoses, conditions, and concerns maintained within the EHR to support continuity of care. Keeping it accurate and up to date is a certified-EHR function and a quality concern, since stale entries can mislead clinical decision support. It is often coded using SNOMED CT and ICD-10-CM.

Project Management. The application of knowledge, skills, tools, and techniques to project activities to meet defined objectives within constraints of scope, schedule, cost, and quality. In healthcare IT it coordinates implementations, upgrades, and integrations across clinical and technical stakeholders. Common processes span initiation, planning, execution, monitoring and controlling, and closing.

QHIN (Qualified Health Information Network). Under TEFCA, a network that has been designated to connect and exchange health information nationwide according to the Common Agreement. QHINs serve as the backbone that links HIEs, providers, payers, and other participants for trusted, nationwide data exchange. They are central to operationalizing TEFCA's vision of universal connectivity.

RACI. A responsibility-assignment matrix that clarifies roles by labeling each task or deliverable as Responsible (does the work), Accountable (ultimately answerable), Consulted (provides input), or Informed (kept updated). It prevents confusion and gaps in ownership on cross-functional projects. RACI is widely used in healthcare IT implementations involving many stakeholders.

RFP (Request for Proposal). A formal procurement document soliciting detailed proposals from vendors to meet defined requirements, used during system selection. It specifies functional, technical, security, and support requirements and evaluation criteria, enabling structured comparison of bids. The RFP process supports objective, defensible vendor decisions.

Risk Analysis. A systematic process required by the HIPAA Security Rule to identify potential threats and vulnerabilities to ePHI, assess their likelihood and impact, and determine appropriate safeguards. It is the foundation of a security-management program and must be conducted and updated periodically. Failure to perform an adequate risk analysis is a frequent cause of enforcement actions.

RPM (Remote Patient Monitoring). The use of connected devices to collect physiologic and health data—such as blood pressure, glucose, weight, or heart rhythm—from patients outside traditional clinical settings and transmit it to care teams. RPM supports chronic-disease management and reimbursable virtual care. It generates large data volumes requiring integration, governance, and security attention.

RxNorm. A standardized terminology for clinical drugs and drug-delivery devices, produced by the National Library of Medicine, that normalizes names across pharmacy and EHR systems. It enables interoperable exchange of medication data and links to other drug vocabularies. RxNorm is a named medication standard within USCDI.

SaMD (Software as a Medical Device). Software intended for one or more medical purposes—such as diagnosis, treatment, or prevention—that performs these functions without being part of a hardware medical device. SaMD, including many AI-driven tools, may be subject to FDA regulation depending on risk. CAHIMS candidates should recognize that not all health software is SaMD, but clinical-decision and diagnostic algorithms often are.

SDLC (Systems Development Life Cycle). A structured framework describing the phases of building and maintaining an information system, commonly including planning, analysis, design, development, testing, implementation, and maintenance. It provides discipline and traceability for healthcare IT projects, whether implementing or configuring systems. Agile and waterfall are alternative ways of moving through these phases.

SNOMED CT (Systematized Nomenclature of Medicine—Clinical Terms). A comprehensive, multilingual clinical terminology providing standardized codes and relationships for clinical findings, procedures, body structures, and more. It enables precise, computable documentation and is widely used for problem lists and clinical data exchange. As a reference terminology, it supports semantic interoperability across systems.

TEFCA (Trusted Exchange Framework and Common Agreement). A national framework established under the 21st Century Cures Act to enable secure, nationwide health information exchange through a common set of principles and a legal agreement. It connects networks via designated QHINs to create a "network of networks." TEFCA aims to make trusted interoperability the default across the country.

Telehealth. The delivery of healthcare services and clinical information using telecommunications technology, including live video visits, store-and-forward transmission, and remote monitoring. It expands access, particularly for rural and mobility-limited patients, and surged during and after the COVID-19 era. Telehealth raises licensure, reimbursement, privacy, and connectivity considerations.

USCDI (United States Core Data for Interoperability). A standardized set of health data classes and constituent data elements designated by ONC for nationwide, interoperable health information exchange. It specifies which data—such as problems, medications, allergies, and clinical notes—must be exchangeable and references standards like LOINC, SNOMED CT, and RxNorm. USCDI is updated through successive versions to expand the shared data baseline.

WBS (Work Breakdown Structure). A hierarchical decomposition of the total scope of project work into smaller, manageable deliverables and work packages. It clarifies what must be done, supports estimating and scheduling, and helps prevent scope omissions. The WBS is a foundational planning artifact that feeds the project schedule and budget.

Interoperability Standards and Terminologies Quick Reference

Interoperability questions are a reliable presence on the CAHIMS exam because they sit at the intersection of every domain in the guide: clinical systems, data exchange, privacy, and analytics all depend on shared standards. This appendix gives you a one-line orientation to each standard you are likely to encounter. For the exam, you rarely need deep technical knowledge of any single standard. You need to know what category it belongs to (messaging, document, API, terminology, identifier, or framework), what kind of data it carries, and where it is used. Read each entry as "what it is, then where it shows up."

.47 Messaging and Document Exchange Standards

HL7 v2.x. The most widely deployed healthcare messaging standard in the world. It uses pipe-and-hat delimited text messages (segments such as MSH, PID, OBR, OBX) to move discrete events between systems: admissions, discharges, and transfers (ADT), lab orders and results, pharmacy, and billing. Despite being decades old and superseded conceptually by FHIR, v2.x still carries the majority of real-time interface traffic inside hospitals, typically routed through an interface engine.

HL7 v3 and the RIM. A ground-up redesign built on the Reference Information Model (RIM) and XML. It aimed for greater semantic precision but proved complex and saw limited adoption beyond a few use cases. Its main lasting product is the document architecture below. Know it mainly as the conceptual bridge between v2 and FHIR.

HL7 CDA (Clinical Document Architecture). An XML standard for encoding clinical documents so they are both human-readable and machine-processable. The Consolidated CDA (C-CDA) templates define common documents such as the Continuity of Care Document (CCD), discharge summary, and progress note. C-CDA was the backbone of Meaningful Use document exchange and is still required for many certified-EHR transitions of care.

FHIR (Fast Healthcare Interoperability Resources). The modern HL7 standard that models healthcare data as modular "resources" (Patient, Observation, Encounter, MedicationRequest, etc.) exchanged over RESTful web APIs using JSON or XML. **FHIR R4** is the normative, regulation-anchored release that ONC certification and the Cures Act API requirements point to. FHIR is the dominant direction of travel for app-based and API-based interoperability.

SMART on FHIR. A specification that layers OAuth 2.0 authorization and OpenID Connect identity onto FHIR, allowing third-party apps to launch securely from within an EHR (or as standalone patient apps) and request scoped access to data. It is the technical foundation for the app ecosystem that the Cures Act patient- and provider-access rules assume.

Bulk Data / Flat FHIR. A FHIR specification for exporting large population-level datasets (entire patient panels) asynchronously, used for analytics, quality reporting, and payer data exchange rather than single-patient lookups.

Direct messaging (Direct Project). A secure, encrypted, email-like protocol (S/MIME over SMTP) that lets providers send patient information point-to-point using trusted Direct addresses. It is the simplest "push" form of interoperability and is widely used for transitions of care and referrals where a full query-based exchange is unavailable.

.48 Application and Networking Standards

DICOM (Digital Imaging and Communications in Medicine). The universal standard for storing, transmitting, and displaying medical images and their metadata (CT, MRI, X-ray, ultrasound). It governs how imaging modalities, PACS, and viewers communicate. Any question about radiology or image archiving points here.

X12 (ANSI ASC X12). The EDI standard for administrative and financial transactions mandated under HIPAA: claims (837), remittance advice (835), eligibility inquiry and response (270/271), and enrollment. When the topic is billing, payer transactions, or revenue cycle data exchange, X12 is the answer, not HL7.

NCPDP. The standard for retail pharmacy transactions, including electronic prescribing (e-prescribing via SCRIPT) and pharmacy claims. Distinguish it from X12 (medical claims) and HL7 (in-hospital pharmacy orders).

.49 Profiles and Frameworks

IHE profiles (Integrating the Healthcare Enterprise). IHE does not create new standards; it specifies how to combine existing ones (HL7, DICOM, etc.) to solve concrete clinical workflows. Key profiles include XDS (Cross-Enterprise Document Sharing) for document repositories and registries, PIX/PDQ for patient identity cross-referencing and demographic query, and ATNA for audit and node authentication. Recognize IHE as the "how to implement consistently" layer.

USCDI (United States Core Data for Interoperability). A standardized, versioned set of data classes and elements (demographics, problems, medications, lab results, clinical notes, and more) that certified health IT must be able to exchange. USCDI replaced the older Common Clinical Data Set and expands by version (v3, v4, and beyond) under ONC stewardship. It defines *what* data must move; FHIR and C-CDA define *how*.

TEFCA (Trusted Exchange Framework and Common Agreement). The federal framework establishing a "network of networks" for nationwide exchange under a single common agreement. It is operationalized through **QHINs (Qualified Health Information Networks)** — designated organizations that connect to each other so participants can query for data across the country. TEFCA represents the policy-and-governance layer that ties regional HIEs into a national fabric and increasingly supports FHIR-based exchange.

HIE (Health Information Exchange). Both the verb (the act of moving health data) and the noun (an organization, often regional or state-level, that facilitates it). Know the three architectures: centralized (data in a shared repository), federated/decentralized (data stays at the source and is queried), and hybrid.

.50 Reference Terminologies and Code Systems

SNOMED CT. A comprehensive clinical reference terminology covering diagnoses, findings, procedures, body structures, and more. It is designed for encoding the *clinical meaning* of data within the EHR (the "problem list" terminology), supporting decision support and analytics. It is a USCDI-named standard for problems and several other data classes.

LOINC (Logical Observation Identifiers Names and Codes). The universal code system for laboratory tests and clinical observations and measurements — what is being measured (e.g., a specific serum sodium test). LOINC names the *observation*; the result value may be coded in SNOMED CT or reported as a number. Critical for lab interoperability.

RxNorm. The normalized naming system for clinical drugs that links the many proprietary drug vocabularies together, enabling medication data to be exchanged and reconciled across systems. It is the USCDI medication standard and underpins e-prescribing and drug-interaction checking.

ICD-10-CM / ICD-10-PCS. ICD-10-CM is the diagnosis classification used for billing, reporting, and statistics in the United States; ICD-10-PCS codes inpatient procedures. These are *classification* systems optimized for reimbursement and epidemiology, contrasted with SNOMED CT, which is optimized for clinical documentation. Many systems map SNOMED-coded problems to ICD-10-CM for claims.

CPT (Current Procedural Terminology). Maintained by the American Medical Association, CPT codes physician and outpatient procedures and services for billing. Paired conceptually with HCPCS Level II (supplies, drugs, and services not in CPT). When a question concerns coding a *service rendered* for a claim, think CPT/HCPCS.

NDC (National Drug Code). A unique identifier for medication products by manufacturer, product, and package size. It identifies the specific marketed package, used in pharmacy dispensing, claims, and supply chain — distinct from RxNorm, which conveys the clinical drug concept.

CVX and other HHS code sets. CVX codes identify vaccines for immunization records and registries. You may also encounter UCUM for units of measure. Recognize these as narrow, purpose-built vocabularies named within USCDI data classes.

.51 How the Pieces Fit (Exam Framing)

For most exam items, sort each standard into one of these buckets and the answer becomes clear: **messaging** (HL7 v2.x for events, X12 for claims, NCPDP for pharmacy), **documents** (C-CDA), **APIs** (FHIR/SMART on FHIR), **images** (DICOM), **terminologies for meaning** (SNOMED CT, LOINC, RxNorm), **codes for billing** (ICD-10-CM, CPT, HCPCS), **identifiers** (NDC, CVX), and **frameworks/governance** (IHE, USCDI, TEFCA/QHIN, Direct, HIE). A common distractor pattern offers a terminology where a transport standard is needed, or a billing code where a clinical terminology is needed. Read the stem for whether it is asking *how data moves* versus *how meaning is encoded* versus *how a service is billed.*

Key Laws, Regulations, and Agencies Crosswalk

Regulatory and governance content is heavily represented on the CAHIMS exam, and the questions tend to test whether you can match a rule to its purpose and to the agency that administers it. This appendix groups the major U.S. healthcare information laws and regulations, names the responsible agency for each, and contrasts them with one international regime (GDPR) that appears for comparison. Focus on three things per item: what problem the rule solves, who enforces it, and what it requires you (as a healthcare IT professional) to do.

.52 HIPAA and Its Rules (Administered by HHS Office for Civil Rights)

HIPAA (Health Insurance Portability and Accountability Act of 1996). The foundational federal law governing the use, disclosure, and protection of individually identifiable health information held by covered entities and their business associates. The Department of Health and Human Services issued the implementing rules below; the **Office for Civil Rights (OCR)** within HHS enforces the Privacy, Security, and Breach Notification rules and levies civil monetary penalties.

HIPAA Privacy Rule. Establishes national standards for protecting protected health information (PHI) in any form — paper, oral, or electronic. It defines permitted uses and disclosures (notably for treatment, payment, and healthcare operations, or "TPO"), grants individuals rights to access and amend their records and to receive an accounting of disclosures, and requires the "minimum necessary" standard for most disclosures.

HIPAA Security Rule. Sets standards specifically for electronic PHI (ePHI). It requires covered entities to implement **administrative, physical, and technical safeguards**, and is built on the principle of a documented, ongoing **risk analysis and risk management** process. Many safeguards are "addressable" (implement, or document why an equivalent alternative is reasonable) rather than strictly "required." This is the rule most directly relevant to IT security work.

HIPAA Breach Notification Rule. Requires covered entities and business associates to notify affected individuals, HHS, and (for large breaches) the media when unsecured PHI is breached. It defines a breach, the timelines (without unreasonable delay and no later than 60 days for individuals; large breaches of 500+ reported to HHS contemporaneously), and the four-factor risk assessment used to determine whether a breach is presumed.

Business Associate Agreement (BAA). The contract HIPAA requires between a covered entity and any vendor that handles PHI on its behalf (cloud hosts, billing services, IT contractors). Recognize that a BAA extends HIPAA obligations down the supply chain; missing BAAs are a common compliance gap.

.53 Strengthening and Modernizing HIPAA

HITECH Act (2009, part of ARRA). The law that put real teeth into HIPAA and launched the EHR era. It strengthened enforcement and increased penalty tiers, extended direct liability to business associates, created the Breach Notification Rule, and — most consequentially — authorized the **Meaningful Use** incentive program (now Promoting Interoperability) that drove nationwide EHR adoption. When a question links EHR adoption incentives or stronger HIPAA penalties to a statute, the answer is HITECH.

Omnibus Rule (2013). The HHS rulemaking that implemented many HITECH provisions, finalizing business-associate liability and the breach standard. Treat it as the regulatory completion of HITECH rather than a separate law to memorize in detail.

.54 Interoperability, Access, and Information Blocking

21st Century Cures Act (2016). Broad legislation whose health-IT provisions prohibit **information blocking** and mandate patient access to electronic health information through standardized APIs. It directed ONC to define information blocking and its exceptions and to advance app-based access "without special effort."

Information Blocking Rule (ONC). Implements the Cures Act prohibition: actors (providers, health IT developers of certified health IT, and HIEs/HINs) may not engage in practices that interfere with the access, exchange, or use of electronic health information, unless a defined **exception** applies (for example, preventing harm, protecting privacy, security, infeasibility, or content-and-manner exceptions). Penalties and disincentives apply. This is a high-yield exam topic; know that the default is "share unless an exception clearly applies."

ONC (Assistant Secretary for Technology Policy / Office of the National Coordinator for Health IT). The HHS office that administers the **Health IT Certification Program**, defines certification criteria, stewards **USCDI**, and writes the information-blocking regulations. When a rule concerns *certified health IT, data standards*, or *information blocking*, the agency is ONC. (The office now operates within the Assistant Secretary for Technology Policy; either name may appear.)

ONC Health IT Certification Program. The voluntary-but-effectively-required program that tests and certifies EHRs and other health IT against criteria (including FHIR R4 API capability and USCDI support). Providers must use certified technology to participate in CMS incentive and reporting programs.

.55 Payment, Participation, and Program Administration

CMS (Centers for Medicare & Medicaid Services). The HHS agency that pays for and regulates participation in Medicare and Medicaid. CMS administers the programs that financially motivate health-IT adoption and exchange, and sets the conditions facilities must meet to be reimbursed.

Promoting Interoperability Program (formerly Meaningful Use). The CMS program (with separate tracks for hospitals and clinicians, the latter under MIPS) that ties Medicare/Medicaid payment to the meaningful use of certified EHR technology — e-prescribing, exchanging health information, providing patient electronic access, and reporting measures. It is the financial engine behind interoperability adoption and is administered by CMS, distinct from ONC's certification role.

CMS Conditions of Participation (CoPs) and Conditions for Coverage. The health and safety standards facilities must meet to receive Medicare/Medicaid payment. Relevant to health IT are requirements such as electronic event notifications (admission, discharge, transfer notifications to other providers) and patient-access expectations woven into CMS rules. Recognize CoPs as participation prerequisites, not optional best practices.

CMS Interoperability and Patient Access Rules. CMS rules (paralleling ONC's) that require payers and providers to support FHIR-based patient-access and provider-directory APIs and ADT event notifications, extending interoperability obligations to the payer side of the system.

.56 Device, Software, and Safety Oversight

FDA and Software as a Medical Device (SaMD). The Food and Drug Administration regulates software that meets the definition of a medical device — software intended for diagnosis, treatment, or prevention. The Cures Act narrowed FDA's scope so that certain low-risk clinical decision support, administrative, and wellness software is *not* regulated as a device. Know the boundary: software that drives a clinical decision a clinician cannot independently review tends to fall under FDA oversight; software that merely informs does not. The FDA's risk-based framework determines the level of premarket scrutiny.

.57 Cybersecurity Guidance and Frameworks

HHS 405(d) Program and HICP. A public-private effort (named for Section 405(d) of the Cybersecurity Act of 2015) that produced the **Health Industry Cybersecurity Practices (HICP)** publication — voluntary, consensus-based practices for managing the most common cyber threats (phishing, ransomware, loss/theft of devices, insider threats, attacks on connected medical devices, and attacks against network-connected systems). It is guidance, not a mandate, but HHS considers recognized security practices when evaluating enforcement. Treat 405(d)/HICP as the go-to voluntary framework for healthcare cybersecurity.

NIST frameworks (context). The NIST Cybersecurity Framework and NIST SP 800-66 (HIPAA Security Rule implementation guidance) are commonly referenced standards that organizations adopt to structure a HIPAA-compliant security program. Recognize NIST as the source of widely used, non-mandatory frameworks rather than a regulator.

.58 International Contrast

GDPR (General Data Protection Regulation, European Union). The EU's comprehensive data-protection law, included here for contrast with HIPAA. Differences worth knowing: GDPR protects *all* personal data of EU residents (not just health data) and applies to far more organizations than HIPAA's covered entities; it grants stronger individual rights, including data portability and a "right to erasure"; it generally requires an explicit lawful basis (often consent) for processing; and it carries large percentage-of-revenue fines enforced by national Data Protection Authorities, not OCR. The exam may ask you to distinguish HIPAA's sector-specific, U.S. scope from GDPR's broad, rights-centric, extraterritorial reach.

.59 Crosswalk Summary for Quick Recall

When an item names a *rule or program*, map it to the agency: HIPAA Privacy/Security/Breach and HITECH enforcement to **HHS OCR**; certification, USCDI, and information blocking to **ONC**; Promoting Interoperability, Conditions of Participation, and payer-access rules to **CMS**; medical-device software to the **FDA**; voluntary cybersecurity practices to **HHS 405(d)**. When an item describes a *purpose* — protecting PHI confidentiality (Privacy Rule), securing ePHI through safeguards and risk analysis (Security Rule), notifying after a breach (Breach Notification Rule), incentivizing EHR use (HITECH/Promoting Interoperability), forbidding data hoarding (information blocking), or comparing to a broad European regime (GDPR) — work backward to the rule and then to the agency. That two-step (purpose to rule to agency) handles the large majority of regulatory items.

Exam-Day Strategy and the Two-Week Final Review

You have learned the material across the chapters of this guide. This appendix is about converting that knowledge into a passing score under timed, computer-based conditions. The CAHIMS is an entry-level credential, and the exam rewards calm, systematic test-taking as much as raw recall. The first half covers tactics for the testing session itself; the second half is a concrete 14-day final-review plan keyed to the guide's domains.

.60 Know the Format Before You Sit Down

The CAHIMS is a computer-based exam of roughly **115 scored multiple-choice items delivered in a two-hour window**, often with a small number of additional unscored pretest items mixed in that do not count toward your result. You cannot tell which items are unscored, so treat every question as if it counts. Two hours for about 115 scored questions works out to a little over a minute per item on average — comfortable if you keep moving, tight if you let any single question consume you. Confirm the exact current item count and timing in your official candidate handbook before exam day, because these parameters are periodically updated, and arrive early enough to complete check-in without rushing.

.61 Time Management

Set internal checkpoints. Rather than watching the clock per question, set a few milestones: roughly one quarter of the questions answered by the 30-minute mark, half by 60 minutes, three quarters by 90 minutes. If you are behind a checkpoint, pick up the pace and lean harder on elimination; if you are ahead, you have earned time for the flagged items.

Never let one item eat your budget. If a question is taking more than about 90 seconds, make your best elimination-based choice, flag it, and move on. A blank or skipped question helps no one; a flagged answered question costs you nothing and can be revisited. The single most common avoidable failure mode is spending five minutes on one hard item and then rushing the last twenty.

Answer every question. There is no penalty for guessing on the CAHIMS, so no item should be left blank. Before you submit, confirm there are no unanswered questions.

.62 Reading Scenario Stems

Many CAHIMS items are short scenarios — a situation involving a hospital, a project, a security incident, or a data exchange — followed by a question. The scenario can contain detail designed to distract.

Read the actual question first, then the scenario. Glance at the final sentence (the "stem" question) before wading through the setup, so you know what you are hunting for as you read.

Identify your role and the goal. Scenarios usually cast you as an analyst, project team member, or coordinator. Ask: what is this person being asked to *do or decide*, and what is the desired outcome (compliance, patient safety, project success, data integrity)? The correct answer almost always serves the patient, the organization's compliance posture, or sound project methodology — rarely the shortcut.

Strip the noise. Names, dates, and incidental numbers are often filler. Underline (mentally) the facts that change the answer: the type of data, the phase of a project, the regulation implicated, the stakeholder affected.

.63 Handling Distractors and Answer Choices

Eliminate first, then choose. On any item you are unsure of, identify and remove the choices you know are wrong before deciding among what remains. Cutting four options to two roughly doubles your odds even if you must then guess.

Watch for the partly-true distractor. The most dangerous wrong answer is one that is true in isolation but does not answer *this* question, or is true but not the *best* response. Reread the stem against your chosen answer to confirm it actually addresses what was asked.

Beware absolutes and extremes. Options containing "always," "never," "all," or "none" are frequently (not invariably) wrong in a field full of "it depends" and "addressable" requirements. Conversely, measured language ("generally," "should," "is typically") often signals a defensible answer.

Do not over-think with outside knowledge. Answer from the standard frameworks this guide teaches — HIPAA, project management fundamentals, the data lifecycle, interoperability categories — rather than an edge case from personal work experience. The exam tests the consensus model, not your shop's local workaround.

.64 "BEST," "FIRST," and "MOST" Stems

A large share of CAHIMS items ask for the *best*, *first*, *most appropriate*, or *most important* action, which means **more than one option is correct** and you must rank them.

For "FIRST" or "NEXT" questions, think in sequence: what step logically precedes the others? In security incidents, containment and following the incident-response plan generally precede notification. In projects, planning and stakeholder analysis precede execution. In a privacy event, verifying whether a breach actually occurred precedes external reporting. Choose the earliest correct action, not the most dramatic one.

For "BEST" or "MOST APPROPRIATE" questions, all options may be plausible; select the one that most fully and safely accomplishes the goal with the least risk and the best alignment to standards. Patient safety, regulatory compliance, and data integrity outrank speed and convenience.

For "MOST IMPORTANT" questions, weigh impact and risk: the answer is usually the choice that, if neglected, causes the greatest harm.

When you see these capitalized qualifiers, slow down for a few extra seconds — they are the markers of a ranking question, and the test writers expect you to discriminate between good and best.

.65 Flag-and-Review Discipline

Use the exam software's flag feature deliberately. Flag any item where you guessed, felt unsure, or noticed a term you might recall later — but **answer it before flagging** so nothing is left blank. Reserve your final minutes for a focused pass over flagged items only; do not re-read the entire exam. When revisiting, change an answer only if you find a concrete reason (you misread the stem, recalled a fact, or another question jogged your memory). Random second-guessing tends to convert right answers to wrong ones; trust your first reasoned choice unless evidence overturns it.

.66 Mental and Physical Readiness

Sleep matters more than a final all-nighter; an alert mind reads stems accurately and resists distractors. Eat beforehand, hydrate, and for an in-person testing center, plan travel with a buffer. For a remote-proctored exam, test your equipment, clear your room, and verify your ID and check-in requirements in advance. During the exam, if anxiety spikes, take three slow breaths and return to your elimination method — the structure of the process steadies you when recall feels shaky.

.67 The Two-Week (14-Day) Final Review Plan

This plan assumes you have already studied the full guide and are now consolidating. Adapt the day allocations to your weakest domains as revealed by your practice scores. Each day pairs targeted review with active recall (self-quizzing) rather than passive re-reading, because retrieval practice is what moves knowledge into exam-ready memory.

Day 1 — Diagnostic and planning. Take a full-length timed practice test under realistic conditions. Score it by domain. Rank your domains from weakest to strongest; this ranking governs how much time you give each topic over the next twelve days. Note every missed item's *reason* (didn't know, misread, careless), not just the right answer.

Day 2 — Healthcare environment and organizations. Review the structure of the U.S. healthcare system: provider types and care settings, payers, accreditation bodies, and the roles of HHS, ONC, CMS, FDA, and OCR (use Appendix E as your crosswalk). Self-quiz on which agency owns which rule.

Day 3 — Health information systems. Review core clinical and administrative systems: EHR, CPOE, CDS, pharmacy, LIS, RIS/PACS, registration/ADT, and revenue cycle. Be able to state each system's primary function and the data it produces.

Day 4 — Data, information, and analytics. Review the data lifecycle (capture, storage, use, archive, destruction), data quality dimensions, structured versus unstructured data, databases, data warehouses, and basic analytics and reporting concepts. Practice distinguishing data from information from knowledge.

Day 5 — Interoperability and standards. Drill Appendix D until you can bucket every standard into messaging, document, API, terminology, identifier, or framework, and state where each is used. This is high-yield; spend the full day if interoperability was weak on Day 1.

Day 6 — Privacy, security, and compliance. Review the HIPAA Privacy, Security, and Breach Notification rules in depth; the three categories of safeguards; risk analysis; and the difference between privacy, security, and confidentiality. Re-read Appendix E's HIPAA and HITECH sections and self-quiz on breach timelines and the minimum-necessary standard.

Day 7 — Mid-point practice test. Take a second full-length timed test. Compare domain scores against Day 1 to confirm your weak areas are improving. Re-plan the remaining days toward any domain still lagging.

Day 8 — Cybersecurity and risk. Review threats (phishing, ransomware, insider, device), controls (access control, encryption, audit logging, authentication), the 405(d)/HICP practices, and incident-response sequencing. Practice "FIRST step in an incident" style questions.

Day 9 — Project and change management. Review project lifecycle phases, scope/time/cost constraints, stakeholder management, requirements gathering, testing, go-live and support, and the basics of system development life cycle. Drill "FIRST/NEXT" sequencing questions, which cluster here.

Day 10 — Leadership, governance, and workflow. Review IT governance, data governance, organizational change, training and adoption, workflow analysis and redesign, and the human factors of system implementation. Connect these to why systems succeed or fail.

Day 11 — Quality, regulation, and reimbursement. Review quality measurement and reporting, the Promoting Interoperability program, Conditions of Participation, value-based care concepts, and how reimbursement models shape IT priorities. Tie programs back to the administering agency.

Day 12 — Targeted weak-area drilling. Spend the entire day on your one or two weakest domains as identified by the Day 7 test. Use active recall and re-work every previously missed item until you can explain *why* the right answer is right and each distractor is wrong.

Day 13 — Final full-length practice test and tactics rehearsal. Take a last timed test, deliberately practicing the tactics in this appendix: question-first reading, elimination, checkpointing, and flag-and-review. Aim to finish with time to spare. Review only the items you missed; do not cram new material.

Day 14 — Light consolidation and rest. Do a light pass over your summary notes, Appendices D and E, and your personal list of facts that keep slipping. Stop studying by mid-afternoon. Confirm your exam logistics — location or remote check-in, identification, start time, and what you may bring. Prioritize sleep. You have prepared systematically; trust the process.

.68 Final Reminders

Bring your knowledge, your tactics, and your composure. Read every stem for what it actually asks, eliminate before you choose, respect the "BEST/FIRST/MOST" markers, answer every item, and reserve your final minutes for flagged questions only. The CAHIMS rewards the steady, methodical candidate, and the fourteen-day plan above is designed to make you exactly that.

www.ingramcontent.com/pod-product-compliance
Lightning Source LLC
LaVergne TN
LVHW062028051126
851858LV00005B/113
* 9 7 9 8 2 5 9 5 0 2 4 6 8 *